Becoming BioQuantum™
Part 1: Activate Cell Ascension

Jewels Arnes: Author
Cerena Lauren: Co-Author

"It takes courage and commitment to choose to come out of the Matrix. We are not meant to do this alone. Together we can shift what it is to be human and awaken to the New Human Experience." – Jewels

Becoming BioQuantum™

ALL RIGHTS RESERVED: No part of this book may be reproduced, stored, or transmitted, in any form, without the express and prior permission in writing of Crossroads Publishing, LLC. This book may not be circulated in any form of binding or cover other than that in which it is currently published. This book is licensed for your personal enjoyment only. All rights are reserved. Crossroads Publishing, LLC does not grant you the right to resell or distribute this book without prior written consent of both Crossroads Publishing, LLC and the copyright owner of this book. This book must not be copied, transferred, sold or distributed in any way.

Disclaimer: Neither Crossroads Publishing, LLC, or our authors will be responsible for repercussions to anyone who utilizes the subject of this book for illegal, immoral or unethical use.

The views expressed herein do not necessarily reflect that of the publisher. This book or part thereof may not be reproduced in any form, stored in a retrieval system, or transmitted in any form by any means-electronic, mechanical, photocopy, recording or otherwise-without prior written consent of the publisher, except as provided by United States of America copyright law.

This book is authentically written and designed. The authors have approved the final PDF of this book and the formatting.

No part of this book may be used for anything AI related, training, creating, etc.

Crossroads Publishing, LLC—620-204-1710

ISBN: 979-8-9926485-5-3

Author Jewels Arnes

Co-author Cerena Lauren

Cover and Graphis by Angela Torres

Edited by Cerena Lauren and Tonya Andrews

Dedications

To my daughters, Sage and Rose —

You are the light that reminds me of the infinite beauty and power that lives within us all.

Your wisdom, your courage, and your grace inspire me to dream bigger, love deeper, and rise higher.

May you always remember you hold the truth of the universe within you and your presence in this world is a gift beyond measure.

This book is a blueprint of human evolution — a future I see because I witness it in you.

- Jewels Arnes

For my son, Joshua, the Light of my life. You continue to inspire with your brilliance, your sensitivity and especially your heart.

– Cerena Lauren

Becoming BioQuantum™
Activate Cell Ascension & Learn to Live as Frequency

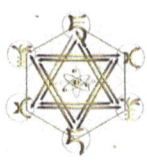

"There is Woo-Woo and there is Woo-True. This is Woo-True." -Luke Story Lifestyle Podcast Interview, "The Quantum Intelligence of DNA"

"There are people who have a deep vibe and a connection to things and people can tell they walk around in another state than most people do. Jewels is one of those people." – Dave Asprey, The Human Upgrade Interview, "Where Quantum Science Meets Spirituality"

"As a result of this work, I am organically moved to participate in my own life at a different level. I am delightfully experiencing upgraded personal growth and self-discovery and have a deeper purpose to my existence as an evolved human being. Daily, I choose to challenge myself, to sharply observe and then determine how I authentically make decisions and interact with others. I engage with the world from different levels of Consciousness knowing that choices can always be upgraded to my next inspired action. Most importantly, I've come to own a deeper sense of my inner Divine nature and most often consciously navigate interactions with the energy and frequency of Divine Love. I am trusting my intuition which I know are whispers of Divine Guidance. I keep looking up, moving forward, co-creating with God and actually being the Creation. This is a very, very big deal!" – Trish

"I am not the same being I was before these teachings. I am continually shifting in my Consciousness, connection, clarity and confidence. The knowledge and tools that Jewels shares are keys to be the creator beings we came to be. Jewels led us through the foundational principles that enable us to transcend the programs of our mind and move into the realms of creating our next in our now. With practice, practice, practice, the results are beyond my wildest imagination. I highly recommend this book to anyone feeling called!" – Ellen

"Enormous Thank You for a frightfully sublime experience. It felt as though I'd gotten on a different flight/destination than I'd imagined. There are no words in my lexicon to express where I am seeking to land right now. I can only speculate how exceptional yet disturbingly familiar it is. What makes a human being special? You're an incredibly delightful expression of its emergence." – Liz

"I am forever grateful for this Ascension University, this school of mastery. My life has never been the same since I made the discovery that my looping behaviors were a plethora of programs running by default in the operating system of my cellular makeup. My experience of life was a printout of my limiting beliefs. Through this work I have learned to tap into my full potential by shifting my Consciousness/attention inward and aligning with the innate truth of who I am. I AM Source Intelligence! Now in my 89th year of life, I am more excited about living than ever before. I have more energy, more vitality and more curiosity as to what new perspective, new revelation will be shown to me as I continue to raise in Consciousness." – Sandy

"Jewels' work has given me access to everything I've ever wanted and to a way of living I didn't know was possible. For years I had intuited that life could be different and that the spiritual journey could be more fun and easier. All my years of spiritual work had left me looping in cycles of clearing, wanting and frustration. And then I found Jewels. Hallelujah! Jewels offers a way out of not only the endless cycles of self-improvement, but a way out of the Matrix altogether. Once I found Jewels' work, everything changed. I finally learned how to let go of wanting everything I didn't have. And then like magic, everything I'd ever wanted (and more) began flowing into my life. If you open your heart to what Jewels teaches, this will be the last book on spirituality you ever have to buy." – Rebecca

How To Use This Book as An Ascension Tool

The BioQuantum book is the process of ascending on a molecular level and learning to live as Frequency. You will have the experience of this consciously when using the tools and activations. This work is designed to bring your mind, body and reality into higher Frequencies. You will see an area for "Notes" at the end of each chapter. You are invited to reflect on your understanding of the materials and write down your insights.

After completing the book, you will have a reference point to how much you shift in Consciousness the next time you go through the book. You will find your understanding of what it is to "Live as Frequency" has elevated to a higher state. This Technology is activating your DNA even when you are unaware of it. Writing out your thoughts and experiences offers you a reference of the shift and will allow you to see just how far you have come in a short period of time.

Forward

The book you are about to read contains the most life-transforming and empowering information of the 21st Century. No longer are we at the mercy of being "victims" of our genetic makeup or hereditary programming, but we are capable of changing our perceptions and changing the outcome of our genetics with what is now known as epigenetics. We are also capable of moving beyond what we ever thought possible and becoming Super Human or BioQuantum!

By opening our awareness to the God Source Frequency that resides in all of us, in every cell and DNA particle, we can advance our physical reality into something extraordinary. We can shed the belief that we are all destined to "grow old, become ill and die." And instead, we can take the human body into new realms and express it in extraordinary and Super Human ways.

Jewels Arnes has remarkable inner sight and has used it to make the world a better place. Her innate abilities to listen to Higher Guidance have allowed her to develop many high-vibrational products and teachings that are indeed pathways to New Earth, to a new Science, to a new way of operating with our connection to Spirit and Higher Selves.

Jewels started her walk with Spirit at the age of 16 when she had a chance encounter with a woman who saw her gift as a "seer." Through the synergy of connecting with her soul family, she was revealed a method to transform Cellular Intelligence.

With over 30 years in Vibrational Healing and multiple accreditations, Jewels developed her Super Power of tracing energy patterns to find the beliefs or programs that keep us in the cycle of aging and disease. She's created BioQuantum delivery systems as a pathway to shifting from molecular to Frequency. These cutting-edge methods lead us to finding the true power of Becoming BioQuantum™!

Developing a delivery system for people to receive the Frequencies that are advancing the DNA, Jewels started her journey into creating outside molecular structure. This then evolved into a revolutionary method to not only support cells to move beyond limiting beliefs but give people the power to heal themselves. Wanting to bring about groundbreaking changes in DNA Intelligence, Jewels focuses on awakening the next in human evolution by teaching her step-by-step methods to those who feel the calling to enhance the human experience.

Jewels fully stepped into co-creation with her Divine when she heard the message, "Break the God Code. Divine Intelligence is held in your DNA." At that moment, the Jewels felt free. She moved through many trials and errors as she found herself reimagining what it is to be human. It didn't take long for Jewels to tap into creating with Source through abstract Frequency. In this Space, Jewels created a platform that is changing what it means to be human. She finds that unity, oneness and uplifting others is the pathway to creating the Advanced Human Experience.

As the platform evolves, all who choose to be a part of this beautiful collaboration tap into a Frequency that is undeniable! Unity in creation, the pathway to a New Earth is truly magical! Jewels is dedicated to bringing in the energy sequences needed to raise the Frequency of the human experience one cell at a time.

When you read and apply the techniques in this book, you will feel empowered and ALIVE in this world. And THAT is well worth the read as you truly are becoming a New Earth Leader!

~ Lauren Ellis Galey, Founder, New Earth One Network

Note to the Reader

"It takes courage and commitment to choose to come out of the Matrix. We are not meant to do this alone. Together we can shift what it is to be human and awaken to the New Human Experience.

This collaboration is only part of the equation. It is time to do what we came here to do! Are you ready to come out of illusion to create change from within the masses? It takes intentional collaboration, sovereignty, and a willingness to expand beyond the collective. It takes awareness and commitment to move into the space of Universal Consciousness and awaken to your fullest potential.

I honor you for choosing to take the journey into the unknown and navigate the awakening of the Quantum Body. I welcome you to your NEXT and I am here to hold space for your continued evolution. If you are ready to tap into awakening to your highest potential, I am here for you with full commitment to guide you even further than you currently dream to go.

Are you ready to become who you came here to be? The Quantum Human design is in creation. Your Brilliance matters in the world. It is time to connect to the miracle pattern and become 100% Human Potential. I welcome you with open arms and invite you to connect deeply with your Soul purpose." ~Jewels

Introduction

Evolution Technology is groundbreaking telepathic Technology that shifts Consciousness to a cellular level using DMT™ Frequencies. It awakens an Intelligence within you that decodes molecular technology or dormant DNA Codes. This organic Technology is the foundation of the evolved human experience and holds the highest human potential.

You are about to learn about and remote view the software that is running through your cells. You are invited to upgrade to the potential, you on a soul level, know you hold. To access Evolution Technology that shifts the identity of the cells by activating a delivery system to Source or Universal Intelligence. The body learns to shift beyond programmed reality. You become the Quantum Body or Advanced Human.

No religious affiliation

The terms "God, Source and Divine" are not affiliated with religion or created in a reality that holds form. **God**, in relation to this work, is an Intelligence, a Universal God, a Frequency, 963 Hz. to be exact. It is a spatial concept that refers to Frequency and Vibration to assist one on one's personal journey of awakening human potential. It refers to a state of Consciousness connected to pure Source Intelligence.

Contents

How To Use This Book As An Ascension Tool v
Forward vi
Note To The Reader: ix
Introduction: x
Chapter 1: Human Potential 1
Chapter 2: Spiritual Discipline 11
Chapter 3: The 1st Pyramid Of The Evolution Technology 20
Chapter 4: Ascension Through The Light Bodies 29
Chapter 5: The Evolution Technology: Learning The Symbols Of Lu, Sca, 33 52
Chapter 6: The 7 Elements 58
Chapter 7: The God Equation (The God Sphere) 97
Chapter 8: Intuitive Powers: Using Your Divine Intuitive Power Blueprint 105
Chapter 9: Use Your Intuitive Skills 120
Chapter 10: Consciousness Is Creating Your Reality 131
Chapter 11: Awakening The Quantum System 141
Chapter 12: Breaking The God Code: The Inversion Of The Cells 156
Chapter 13: Creating The Quantum Body 167
Chapter 14: Consciously Awakening The Quantum Body 179
Chapter 15: Using The Frequency Of DMT™ 196
Chapter 16: Hourglass Method: Learning To Manifest In Abstract Frequency 225
Chapter 17: 33-Day Evolution Technology 237
Chapter 18: Upgrading Human Potential Through Body Chemistry 278
Glossary 293

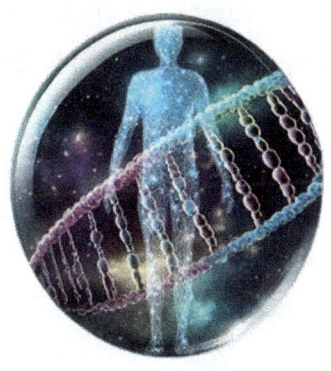

Chapter 1: Human Potential

Evolution Technology is held in the foundation of DNA Intelligence, DMT™. It is the Frequency of 963 Hz. of empowerment that holds the wisdom of the Ascended Human. It teaches you to expand Consciousness beyond your limitations of programmed reality or the programmed body.

Once you realize that you have a choice in how you experience the body, everything changes. You can remain in the looping cycle of age and disease, or you can choose to awaken the Quantum Body. Inside your DNA is the transcribed Intelligence of Source Intelligence.

Using Evolution Technology allows you to tap into the Advanced Intelligence of the DNA. You can see it like a gene code of evolution. It is a gateway to becoming conscious and allows you to actively participate in the evolution of your body. You are invited to take the journey into advancing human potential. This book is for you who desire to awaken and retrieve your birthright as the NEXT in Human Evolution.

Biohacking is one of the greatest frontiers for those looking to master the human body. Understanding the body only biologically is as limiting as only diving deep into the mind.

The intellect will not take you there. To truly become 100% Human Potential, you must move beyond the limitations of the mind. Because of how you access information, you currently only use about 10% of your potential.

The question becomes how to access the 90% of potential that is lying dormant. You must shift everything you think you know and turn it **"inside out."** Because the information you receive from your environment is in duality or is observed through a filter, it is the very programming you are trying to break free from.

You have the ability to move from observation into an expression of Frequency that holds an Intelligence. To neutralize the information, you must remove the ego's experience and replace it with the expression of DNA Intelligence or DMT™. You become the Intelligence of the Body, not the mind. Until you shift from observation of your reality, you remain in the looping cycle of life and death.

Jewels' Story:

"In 2013, I injured my spine. After an unsuccessful surgery, I was devastated. I thought I would be in severe pain and have limited use of my left arm for the rest of my life. As a BioQuantum practitioner, I knew my body had the power to heal. I had an innate "knowing" that I could heal instantly.

One day, while I was doing my daily meditation practice, I spoke out loud, "Divine, if this is how I am supposed to live for the rest of my life, I will make peace with that.

But if You have something else in mind for me, now would be a great time to show me what that is." I went into a deep state of Consciousness; my neck began to pop, and a huge rush of energy ran down my spine. It was like an electric light show. Every cell in my body lit up. In that moment, I healed instantly.

This began my obsession with DNA Intelligence. Your DNA contains the other 90% of your potential, including the ability to heal instantly. So, my journey as a BioQuantum practitioner shifted from focusing on the brain to attuning to the body's Intelligence, specifically the DNA. What I have since discovered is groundbreaking. You hold the ability to tap into a Telepathic Technology that reprograms limiting belief systems on a cellular level. These limitations are your experience of the body as it is."

Cerena's Story:

"I began my journey with the Becoming BioQuantum™ platform about five years ago. Along this path, I have released unconscious survival patterns and continue to heal and youth my being as I discover my Divine within. I let go and reorder my life as I evolve and claim the brilliance that I AM. I release people, places and things which no longer fit my expression as a conscious being committed to Ascension.

I AM forever grateful to Jewels for being the conduit for these profound teachings. I acknowledge the Divine for partnering with me to articulate this material in such a way as to invite you, the reader, along on a journey of ultimate self-discovery to become 100% Human Potential."

The Invitation:

The body is the most advanced technology there is. When you reprogram the cells to shift out of the looping cycle of age and disease, an Intelligence awakens within you. This organic technology is the foundation of the evolved human experience, the awakening of the Quantum Body.

You have the ability to turn on DMT™ codes and become 100% Human Potential. Using DMT™ Frequency, you begin to decode molecular technology. You hold an innate "knowing" that there is more to you than what you are experiencing.

So why reprogram the cells and not the mind? Consciousness is stored in the electrons of the body. Science is showing that all your organs have Consciousness, just like the brain.

The only reason you "think" Consciousness is the brain is because the ego identifies as thought. The ego is the part of you that is separate from the body because it needs observation to exist. You can reprogram the cells to bypass the limited programming of the conscious and subconscious mind.

What if the answer to becoming 100% Human Potential is for you to connect to those dormant Codes/DNA Intelligence? To become the expression of the Intelligence stored within you? You can perceive matter with your mind, but you will only experience the Intelligence of your innate being by consciously tapping into information only found on a cellular level. Just because you don't understand something, just because you can't prove it scientifically, does not mean it's not true.

Material science is not able to see the truth of what it is to be the Ascended Human. Science doesn't have all the answers. Theories continue to be proven wrong. This will continue until a shift from observation of programmed reality in the Quantum Field is replaced by expression through the Intelligence stored inside you.

Feel into it. If you are receiving information from the observation of your reality, you are observing the very loop from which you are trying to break free. No matter how far into the Quantum Field you explore, it is still the Matrix.

When you turn on your DNA Technology, you begin to break out of a programmed reality. You break the looping cycle of age and disease. How to become 100% Human Potential is stored within your very design. To shift beyond limitation, you must stop observing what has already been created. To become the Quantum Body, you must move Consciousness into Cellular Intelligence. Consciousness becomes the body.

You have a choice in how you experience the Intelligence of your body. If you loop in the unconsciousness of genetic expression, you experience age and degeneration. You have the power to break through the loop and consciously awaken the transcribed Intelligence stored in the DNA. Your DNA is more powerful than even the most advanced technology.

It is time to live beyond the illusion of aging. To live a life that is uncharted, beyond programmed reality, beyond what every other human has done before you. It is time to take "impossibilities" and bring them into finite abilities. To create the Ascended Human experience!

You have the power to choose to repeat the looping cycle of the body within the Matrix or to open a gateway through DNA Intelligence. Evolution Technology uses DMT™ Frequency to assist you in reaching your highest potential.

Your cells hold an Intelligence beyond what the mind can comprehend. Your cells are the software system of Source Intelligence stored in your DNA Technology. When you reprogram on a cellular level, you shift the very environment that Consciousness exists within. But more accurately, you shift the vessel, *the body,* it is held within. The body then holds a higher Frequency, which allows Consciousness to shift without subconscious interference. This permits the mind to change without needing to understand the Intelligence that is "turning on."

The body shifts first. Your conscious mind follows, attuning to DMT™ Frequency over time. It is a mind-blowing experience when Consciousness hits the Frequency, and you suddenly become aware of information stored in the Intelligence.

When living within the Matrix, or programmed body, you relate to patterns that were created in a looping cycle. These biological conditions and sources of information have been passed down genetically for generations. The cells unconsciously recreate the life and death cycles based on basic primitive tissue.

Through the Evolution Technology, you begin to break the looping cycle of repeated cellular patterning. You awaken an Intelligence that shifts the cells out of primal behavior and into a current of energy in expression of Source Frequency or DMT™. The cells shift from holding and expressing information from their environment.

When this happens, a Frequency creates a complex system or energetic field for Source Intelligence to move online. The body begins to identify as Frequency without reflection. You can see this system as a Technology. This is the Quantum Body. This system or Technology breaks the looping cycle of cellular behavior and human potential begins to evolve to 100% expression of Source Intelligence. You have the ability to activate DNA Frequency to shift the cells into the expression of Source!

You are invited to become aware of your frequency. The higher your energy or vibration, the lighter you feel in your physical, emotional and mental bodies. As wellbeing increases, you experience less discomfort and pain. Your intuitive awareness soars, and you become more connected to the Universe.

Experience:

Practice frequency awareness by holding a stone in your hand. Tune into the center of the stone. Ask what information the stone has for you. What is its frequency pattern? Continue to receive more information. The more you feel into it, the more information will come. The more you practice moving past your initial impression, the more concrete the information that you receive. Practice reading the initial frequency pattern, then go beyond it.

Home Frequency Exercise:

Your Home Frequency is the basic resonance you were born with. Bring your Consciousness into your High Heart, a space just above your physical heart. This is your Quantum Heart or Advanced Heart.

Once you feel you have entered your High Heart, ask if you are there. Do you feel a subtle "yes" or "no?" Just listen, feel, see or experience the Frequency of your High Heart. The more you resonate in the Frequency of your High Heart, the more you will begin to know your Home Frequency.

You can practice your Home Frequency when you are with another person. When that person begins to talk, allow your Home Frequency to touch the outside of the other person's energy field. The auric field is normally about two feet out from the physical body. Notice what you are experiencing. Move back away from the person's field and check how you feel. Is the energy calm? Prickly? Something else?

When you sensitize yourself to the difference in frequency, you create choice. As you turn on the Quantum Body, you will hold a Frequency well above the average human or reality altogether.

Notes

Notes

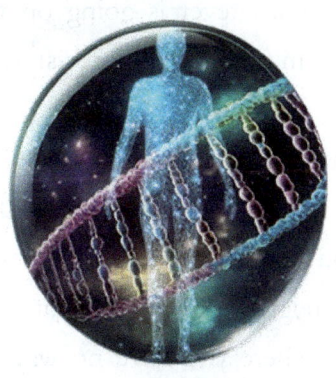

Chapter 2: Spiritual Discipline

Spiritual Discipline, or self-discipline, becomes mandatory if you choose this journey. If you commit to your Ascension! It is to live by self-discipline and not allow emotion, repeated thought or your programming to steer your life.

To make decisions from inner guidance, rather than emotion, is a skill. To decide when, in an emotional response, is to choose from programming. Emotion is expressed through the primal body. Why? Because emotion is a chemical response the body creates as a trigger to its environment.

When creating from emotion, chemical responses of the body interrupt clear, intuitive guidance. When in an emotional reaction, it is best to sit with a decision until the chemical response of the body calms down and you are able to move into stillness. This is also referred to as accessing the High Heart or the Quantum Body.

Most Guidance is the exact opposite of what your ego mind would have you do. This is where Spiritual Discipline becomes critical. Learn to see thoughts, emotions and whatever is going on within as information instead of relying on them to make your decisions.

When operating from mental programming and emotion, you may be inclined to say "no" if a choice seems uncomfortable. In following Source Guidance, you could find yourself in uncharted territory in situations that seem foreign. Following the Intelligence brings you into an abstract Frequency where you have no way of "seeing" your end result. You discover something that you have never created before.

This is when Spiritual Discipline becomes critical. It asks that you surrender to Divine Guidance instead of searching for safety or an answer based on emotions or mental programming. You are invited to stay out of the **"filing cabinet"** of what may have worked for you in the past.

Spiritual Discipline asks you to stay on course no matter how things feel. You may need to take a moment to reset before moving forward. Because something doesn't feel good does not mean it isn't your right course.

To create big change, there may be times of discomfort. Whether because of something you don't want to do or because you have to put in more effort than you expected would be needed, having the discipline to bypass emotion-based decision making frees you to exist beyond programming.

This in itself is Spiritual Discipline! When creating from programming or emotion, you are attempting to cope with stress or discomfort. You have the opportunity to bypass what your mind and emotions tell you, use it as information and stay on course. This is your opportunity to use stress to become aware of programming. Such moments offer the choice to read information and make a conscious decision in your best interest, based on Guidance. When feeling unsure, take a moment to observe whether you are tempted to give up based on your emotions. Notice the difference between taking an inspired action and making your choice based on a potential outcome.

When you choose circumstances or make big choices in order to create a specific end result, most often, you make that decision in order to create an emotion. When you do this, you are destined to repeat the looping cycles of your programming.

The need to feel safe can keep you stuck. If you base a decision on emotion, you are likely to repeat patterns you wish to break. You may wonder why your life isn't changing, why the choices you believed were going to make you happy don't offer the result you expected or were hoping to create.

When making choices from programming and emotion, you repeat cycles and tend to get more of what you already have. This doesn't mean that you're always going to feel amazing, but when triggered, you will clearly see that you've moved into a space of feeling unsafe. A space of primal programming.

You can nurture yourselves in that space and say, **"I feel unsafe right now. I feel afraid. I don't know where this is going to take me, but I also know what it feels like to cave to emotion and programming. I choose to say "yes" to DMT™ Intelligence or Guidance even when I am afraid."**

If you remember the inspirational "yes" that started your journey, you will find it easier to solidify your commitment. Saying "yes" to the Intelligence can bring you out of your comfort zone. You are invited to live in the Unknown, where choices are no longer based on being "safe."

If you find it difficult to move out of emotion or are tempted to release stress in an unhealthy way, try changing things up. Do something like jumping jacks, dancing to high vibe music or taking a walk to bring you back into conscious choice. Choose something to raise your frequency and, once the emotional response or stress has passed, make a conscious choice.

Reflect on your process. Are you making a choice in order to feel comfortable? Are you choosing to do nothing because that feels better? Are you saying "no" when called to say "yes" because you are afraid?

Fear blocks Guidance. Sit with this. Be honest with yourself. What are you being called to say "yes" to? To say "no" to? What inspired action have you begun and are now questioning? Because you aren't seeing the desired outcome or because you are so uncomfortable that you're backtracking?

For example, you receive a download or strong Guidance to take an action. You feel inspired as Source pours into you. You commit to your inspired vision.

Before taking action, take time to sit in your "yes." Invite Source Intelligence to inform you. Know that you are saying "yes" to Guidance beyond your programming. Commit to being the vessel that will bring this inspiration into form. Once you make the commitment, consistently ask to be shown your next right step.

Commit to the next step, no matter how scary or foreign it may seem. Say "yes" and take appropriate action. One day, you will look back on your journey and see the miracle of your creation beyond what you ever imagined.

Attune to the Guidance of DNA Intelligence within you and allow yourself to step into mastery. Honor yourself for choosing this over emotion and programming. In the beginning, this may challenge you. It is, after all, a discipline! The more that you practice, the easier it gets and the more willing you become to "be uncomfortable."

Go back to the moment you received the download to say "yes." Remember that when you follow Spiritual Discipline, you cannot fail. To follow an inspired "yes" from Source, you consistently choose to return to the DMT™ Frequency every time your ego questions or looks for results.

Choose the unknown and manifest something that hasn't been created before. You are here to be a Change Maker! It is time to master and prioritize Spiritual Discipline. When you commit to yourself in this way, you allow yourself to move through the uncomfortable in ways which may surprise you. You solidify your inspired "yes" with commitment.

Begin to live your life in abstract Frequency and allow Source to consistently pour into you. Practice Spiritual Discipline and hone your ability to choose beyond programming and emotion. Rather, see it as information. The more you practice saying "yes" to Guidance, the more the DMT™ Frequency will become your state of being. It will become more real than your programming.

In time, saying "yes" to Source, an Intelligence beyond mental and emotional programming, becomes a way of life. Life becomes your spiritual practice because you become aware of information within old patterns and choose beyond it. You open to the **Miracle Frequency**. To live from there takes Spiritual Discipline!

You are becoming a Change Maker. You keep going when things seem hard. Your strength builds as Source shows you how to rewire the illusion that your experience was ever difficult.

Exercise To Raise Your Frequency:

Place your hands on your heart. Take a deep breath. Invite Source Intelligence/DMT™ into your heart space. Allow the Frequency to inform and infuse your experience beyond programming. Fill yourself with Grace. Feel it move into every cell and molecule of your body. Invite the DMT™ Frequency to amplify within each cell.

Notice your Frequency raise when you invite in Source. As you release resistance, notice how good it feels to surrender to this Frequency. Move your attention to the center of your physical mind. Notice old belief systems that have kept you stuck begin to dissolve.

Repeat, **"I clear the fear of being uncomfortable. I clear, cancel and delete the fear of making the wrong decision. I clear any questioning of my decision. I clear all doubts. I clear, cancel and delete the need to make decisions based on emotional and mental programming. I clear the belief that I am uncomfortable in the Unknown."**

Now state, "**I am willing and able to make decisions based on Guidance through Source Frequency /DMT™. I am willing and able to commit to Spiritual Discipline.** My body knows what it feels like to bypass emotional response and make decisions through an Intelligence beyond programming. I'm willing and able to ask for help when I need strength."

Take a deep breath and allow the DMT™ Frequency to expand your reality. Feel the freedom in the Intelligence within you. Commit to allowing this Frequency to inform your life. Step fully into your power.

It's time to be bold! It is time to become big! You can make big changes by committing to choices based on decisions made outside of your programming. Continue to use Spiritual Discipline as you take action, even when it's uncomfortable. It is time to step into your highest potential!

Notes

Notes

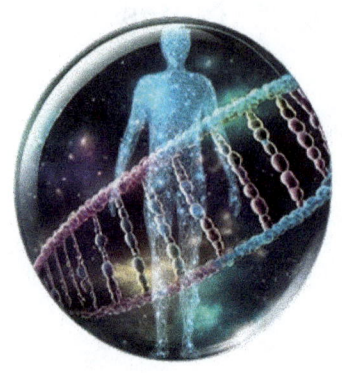

Chapter 3: The 1st Pyramid Of The Evolution Technology

The Body is a Reflection of Consciousness
The 5 States of Consciousness Connected to the 5 Bodies

5 States of Consciousness:
https://becomingbioquantum.com/5LevelsofConsciousness

Learning the 5 States of Consciousness provides a foundation for awareness of where you are existing. As you move into higher States of Consciousness, you begin to notice when you decrease in frequency. Awareness of your State of Consciousness, and its vibrational pattern, creates a choice for you to connect to the highest Frequency and, in time, hold the Frequency of Source Intelligence or
DMT™, 963 Hz.

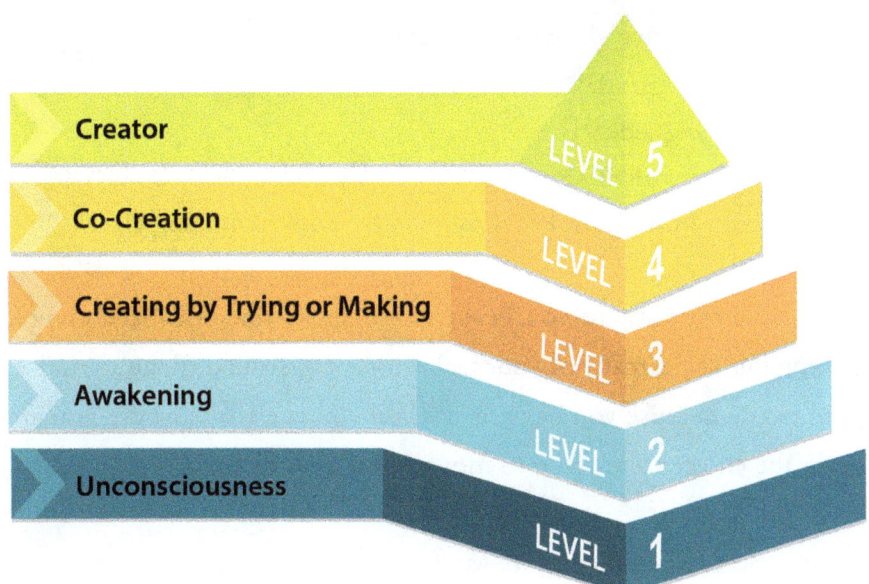

5 Levels of Consciousness

Level 1 State of Consciousness:

You are completely unaware, asleep and unconscious to the idea that you can create choice. You will spend some time here. Ask yourself, **"What am I not seeing?"**

Level 2 State of Consciousness:

You "wake up" and begin to see things coming into your awareness or reality. It is important to stay here and observe in order to move to the 3rd level. This state of Consciousness is where you begin to realize where you have been existing.

You begin to ask important questions such as:

"Am I resisting?"
"Why am I resisting?"

"How is resistance showing up for me?"
"Does this feel good?"
"Does it feel aligned?"
"Do I resonate with this?"
"Do I agree with this, or do I want to agree with something else?"

This is the state where you begin to recognize that you have choice. During this stage, many of your realizations can seem difficult to notice, even harsh, because you begin to view life in a new frequency. You are given the choice to resist or to move to the 3rd State of Consciousness.

Level 3 State of Consciousness:

You begin to move into Creation. You start choosing. This is the Level where you may get stuck trying to *recreate what has already been done*. Instead of creating, you try to make something work.

Existing here can take incredible energy and often seems to go nowhere. This can be because you're not meant to go in the direction you expect and that you are viewing it from the 3rd State of Consciousness, and not from DMT™ or Source Frequency.!

You can likely recall times when you asked, **"Why isn't this working?" "That person did it; why can't I?"** It's because you aren't meant to do it their way. You aren't supposed to do it in a way that you did it before. You are meant to do it from the space of Divine Creation within your heart.

"Trying to make it happen" is also referred to as **"creating form with form."** Manifestation really begins to happen in the 4th and 5th Level of Consciousness.

Level 4 State of Consciousness:

This is the inception point! From here, you are able to sit with the energy you are receiving and allow it to show itself. You begin creating from this space. It's where you **"Listen and do! Listen and do! Listen and do!"**

You don't push, strive, sweat or bleed. You remain in a state of flow and ease. You create according to Divine Design beyond observation of time. You remain open and hold the Frequency. You identify in Frequency more than form. You begin to experience the Quantum Body.

From here, it is easy to recognize when you have fallen back to the 3rd State of Consciousness. It will feel like you are trying hard to make something work. You will notice yourself asking what others did so that you can try to recreate it.

When you notice this, simply invite Source Intelligence into your heart, notice what you are holding there and choose to move back up to the 4th State of Consciousness. This is called **"the inside out process."**

The ability to notice that you are creating through programming demonstrates a huge leap in Consciousness. It is an even bigger accomplishment to hold Consciousness in this higher state. Since programming is no longer running or is not your primary expression, there is very little to identify with. You learn to hold Consciousness in Source Frequency or within the abstract, no form.

Inside out Meditation:
https://becomingbioquantum.com/InsideOutMeditation

Level 5 State of Consciousness:

In the 5th Level of Consciousness, you are in full alignment with Source Intelligence. You become the Creation and the Creator at the same time. Essentially, you create beyond observation, constantly, moment by moment. In this state of being, you become Source Intelligence. There is no gap between listening and doing. You hear before you hear, see before you see, know before you have a thought and feel before you feel anything. DMT™ Intelligence is in full expression, and you exist without observing reality. Reality becomes Source Intelligence. You exist without existing. You become the Advanced Human.

The 1st Pyramid of the Evolution Technology:

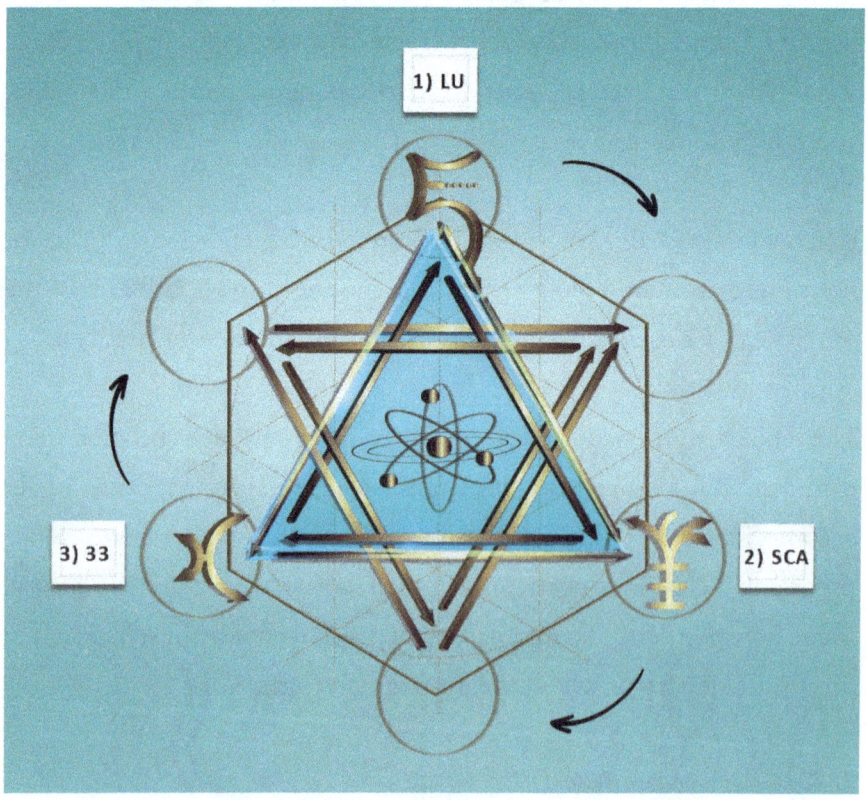

The 5 Levels of the Quantum Body:

1. The **Primal Body** has to do with cell mutation. The body is seen as separate from Consciousness. The 1st Body is the unconscious body and correlates to the 1st Level of Consciousness. The body is not seen as a reflection of self or as a source of information. It's about living out primal programming and reacting to life.

2. The **Chemical Body** expresses the chemical responses of the body and is directly related to the 2nd Level of Consciousness. It can feel like riding on a roller coaster as emotional responses get triggered by programmed stories or thoughts.

3. In the **Neuro/Neural Body** or 3rd Body, programmed responses are signaled to the primal body. Neural pathways are rewired to create change. Form meets form. You are aware that the body holds information, or an Intelligence, and you try to change it through programming or observation.

In the 3rd Level of Consciousness, hardwired programming creates the reality of your body, thoughts, beliefs and emotions. You are triggered by the looping cycles of these programs. Your body is programmed to degenerate. Aging is an epigenetic code.

Epigenetic codes are "turned on" by the environment of a cell when the frequency of the environment is sustained long enough to signal the DNA to turn on that expression. Because these codes can be "turned on," they can be "turned off" by changing the environment. Epigenetics is a result of the first 3 Bodies.

Think about how you "**try**" to rewire the neuro/neural body in order to create change. You may change your mindset. You may even see changes in the way you feel. But you are still living out the 3rd Body. You just changed what program you are running. To become 100% Human Potential, you need to move into the Quantum Body.

4. The 4th Body is the **Quantum Body** and is related to the 4th Level of Consciousness. Thought occurs outside of programming. DMT™ awakens! You begin to identify as an Intelligence beyond what can be seen or studied, creating a Field or Frequency more real than what is observed through programming.

The Quantum Body is your organic Technology that holds a purity of Intelligence stored in your DNA. You can call this Source, Universal Presence, the Divine. It is your innate state of being. The body is already multidimensional. In the first 3 Bodies, you see yourself as matter because of Consciousness held in the programmed body. As you move Consciousness into the 4th Level and actively participate in DMT™ Intelligence, you begin to consciously shift the body into the NEXT of Human Evolution.

5. The 5th Body is the **Advanced Human**, 100% Human Potential. The body and Consciousness assimilate into Oneness. The body becomes DMT™ Intelligence. There is no separation in Consciousness. One being, mind, body and soul, is the Intelligence of Source.

The 5th Body is 100% Human Potential, the Advanced Human. Dormant DNA is fully activated, and you move beyond the Quantum Body. Because this state of being is still revealing itself, it is not yet known exactly what this experience will be.

Notes

Notes

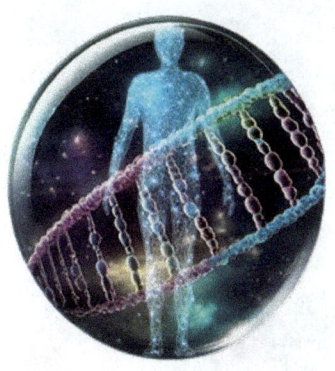

Chapter 4: Ascension Through The Light Bodies

Once the body transforms from form to Quantum, you understand the stages of the Ascended Body or Light Body. The human body will extend five times through vibrational patterns that hold specific knowledge or Intelligence.

Each body exists in space but is not limited within space. The human body will shift on a molecular level five times. Each time it will release density and achieve a higher Frequency. You will progress through 5 different Bodies of Light, shifting from carbon into an organic Technology.

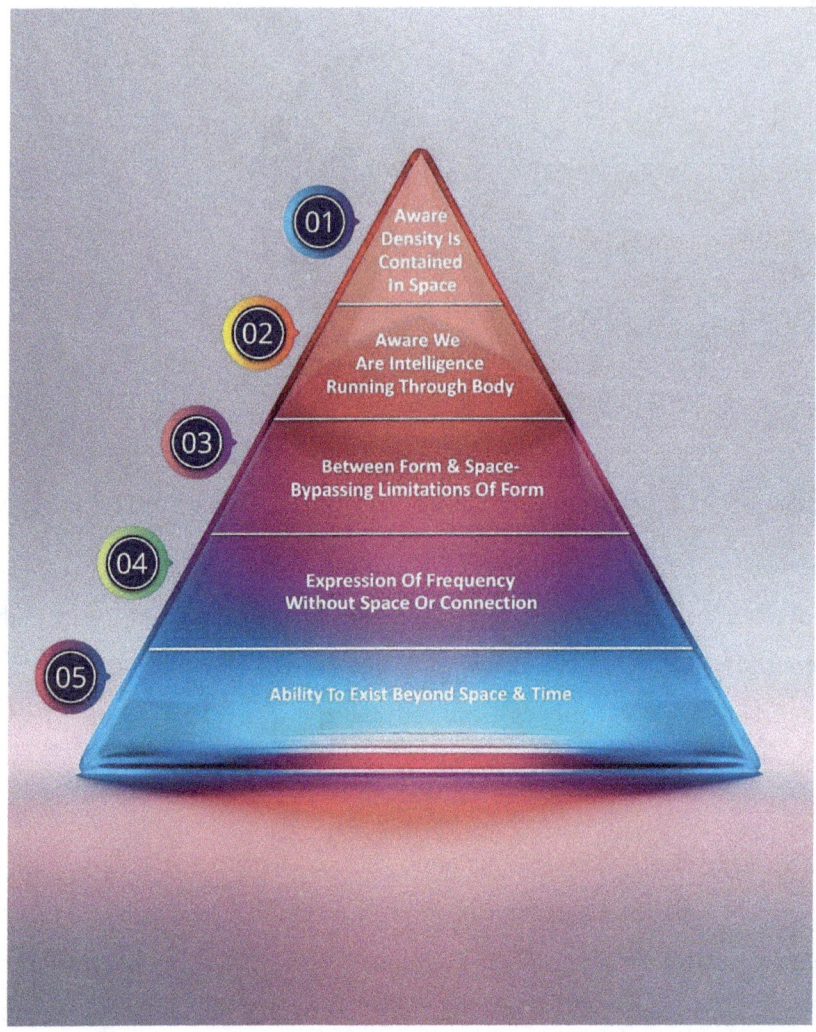

There are 5 Levels of Consciousness connected to each body:

1. Awakening.
2. Seeing the reflection to create choice.
3. Shifting identity by using reflection to create something beyond it.
4. Actively participating as and with Source Intelligence. Awakening through DMT™ Frequency. You are the Quantum Body!

5. Becoming the Intelligence without reflection. You are Source Intelligence in the Advanced Human form.

The body knows or holds Source Intelligence before the mind can comprehend what is being held. There is much information available on the Light Body. For this discussion, see the Light Body as the conscious transition from density to Frequency.

The Light Body is connected to Consciousness. Consciousness shifts as the body shifts. You wake up the body first. The body has the ability to hold an Intelligence, run the software of Source Intelligence and exist beyond programmed reality.

That Intelligence, as it comes online, creates energetic patterns not in the experience of the body now. Depending on what phase of the Light Body you are in, you will experience the body in a different density or release of density.

As you evolve, you will experience moments of less density. As a Wayshower or pioneer in awakening the Quantum Body, you commit to traverse this experience as consciously as possible, so you are able to demonstrate the process to others.

You are in the very vehicle through which you will consciously ascend. Most people spend most of their time between the 1st and 2nd Light Body.

Why 5?

You will go through all 5 Levels of Consciousness in each Level of the Light Body. Each stage begins with awareness. You first have to wake up and see the illusion in order to move to the next Level. You have to be able to hold a Level in expression for long enough in order to shift to the next Level.

For example, when you move into the 4th Light Body, you will still be experiencing some of the 3rd until your cells fully shift into multidimensional form. The 5th Light Body relates to the 5th Level of Consciousness.

1st Light Body

The 1st Light Body is that awakening piece. You've been plugged into a frequency pattern or timeline connected to programmed reality, which creates slow degeneration over time. The programmed body is collective consciousness; it is the consciousness of repeated agreements that create a strong frequency which creates your reality.

Programmed reality or the Matrix is like a computer system that runs unconsciously. Once you wake up to an unconscious program, you have the ability to unplug and shift. In this state, you have awareness that density is contained in space. You break the illusion that the body is the self and that the experience of the body is the truth.

Consciously, you have some idea that the body is holding space. You realize the container that is your Consciousness is the illusion itself. The body is a container with energy that forms space which creates density. The body is the Matrix, created in the illusion of the Super Hologram or your programmed belief systems.

Know that there's more than what you experience in form, beyond the limitations of the body. The goal is to become aware of limitations within the Matrix. To become aware of where in your body you agree to density or programming.

Density is slow moving particle waves. Get to know your spin state and what you're agreeing to. It's about knowing what you're not choosing. You do not have to know what you are choosing differently.

Because the body is a reflection of Consciousness, it shows what needs to be seen in order to advance to a higher Frequency. The body teaches you not to look outside yourself for evidence. If you're caught up in thoughts of "Is this working?" know that you are in reflection and not in the level of Consciousness you will exist in when you move into higher Light Bodies.

In the 1st Light Body, you are also working with the 1st and 2nd Elements: **"I AM Not My Mind. I AM Not My Thoughts."** (The Elements will be further explored in chapter 6.) Your mind is a program of how you define yourself within the Matrix.

If you have mastered the 1st Light Body, you are able to state, **"I am not my body. My body is the experience of the I AM."** You will have completely identified as the I AM that is experiencing the body and no longer claim that the body is who you are. The I AM remains because you still have to have an identity. However, the I AM is identifying with your Soul or Spirit and not the body itself.

This is the stage where the Hydrogen Atom comes online and creates at a higher spin state or Frequency. When you become aware you are not the body, it is your first awakening that cellular structure is in a looping cycle. It creates space between reality, allowing an Intelligence beyond the programming of the body to come in. This allows the body to begin to "turn on" Frequencies that elevate Consciousness and activate the Quantum Body.

2nd Light Body

In this state, you see the concept of existing beyond form, or the body, as a direct reflection of Consciousness. You use reflection to elevate beyond the programming of the body.

Thoughts that program the body are referred to as **"looping cycles."** Consciousness rises so that you are able to see the body as a source of information. You start to bring DMT™ Intelligence into the Quantum Body. The body moves past limitations to expand in Consciousness. The Frequency of Source Intelligence moves into the body. Consciousness has the ability to read belief systems that are connected to the experience of the first three physical bodies. Once you see the beliefs that create limitations in the body, you have the ability to consciously attune to a Frequency that is at a higher state.

If you are in pain or have something of concern in your body, it is the body showing you density or cells in a low spin state or frequency. Particles spin very slowly when connected to the degeneration cycle of the programmed body. When shifted, using Evolution Technology to activate DMT™, their spin state increases. The particles release and start to move into a state where the body identifies itself as Frequency. This brings the cells into the Quantum Field.

The body is the most advanced Technology there is. It is pure Source Intelligence, the Intelligence from which you were created, in expression. You can read belief systems in programmed reality because the body suggests to not limit yourself to programming and instead choose a higher Frequency.

You have the ability to explore just how limitless you are by not agreeing to belief systems. A Frequency of possibility, to exist outside of that limitation, begins to release and move into your body.

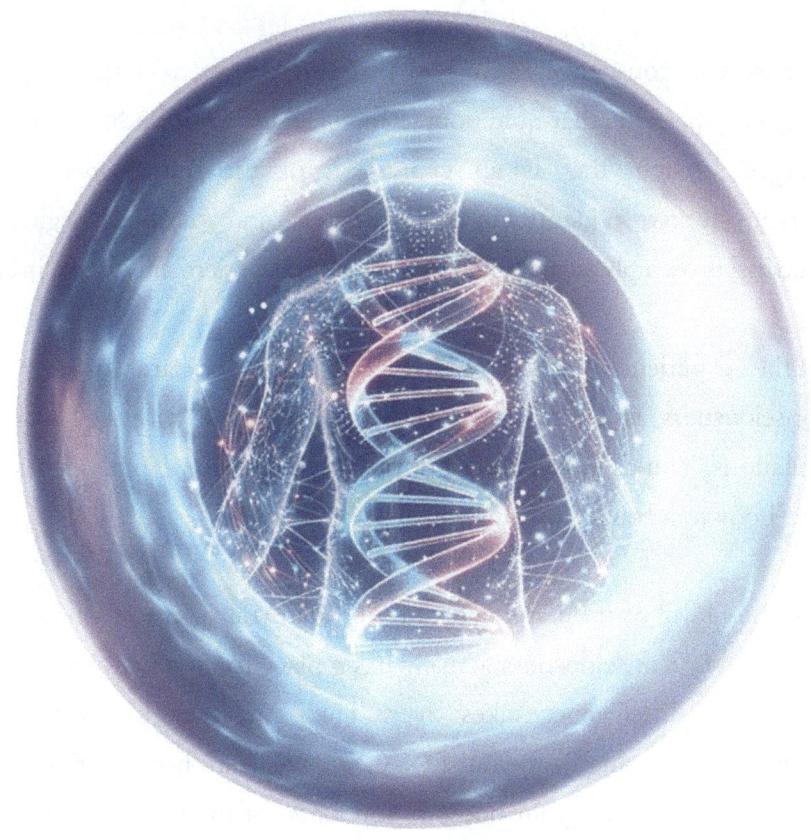

Your body has billions of little energy responses, electrons, hanging out in your body that are not yet activated. This is your Quantum Body. Source Intelligence releases from the DNA and moves into the body. The body begins to identify as the Quantum Body to hold the Frequency.

The Frequency breaking the belief systems creates a new energetic response…and another… and another…which creates an energetic pattern that holds the Intelligence breaking the belief systems. The body begins to attune to the Quantum Body and starts to use these energetic responses to create a bridge between the physical and the Quantum Body. This is your software system, an organic Technology.

Because you consciously attune to this Intelligence, you start to run Frequency patterns that hold Source Intelligence. Your body creates an energetic system that is an expression of this Intelligence. You consciously start to identify in this Intelligence and your body begins to override its own physical limitations to match the energetic system itself.

In the experience of the 2nd Light Body, you are aware that Consciousness is shifting and that your body is moving beyond limitations. You use reflection of physical and emotional experiences of your body to advance in Consciousness.

Your body will turn on and evolve faster than your Consciousness can understand. Consciousness actually has a place to go where limitation leaves, and Intelligence takes over. Think of it as following the Intelligence releasing from your DNA. You will learn how limitless you are. Your mind limits your body. If you let go of thinking through the programmed mind, the body can do so much more.

All limitations of what the body "needs" can go away. For now, it is important to do what you think your body needs. You want to optimize your mitochondria health in this stage of the body's Ascension. You want your body in pristine condition.

Treat your body as the Ascension Vehicle it is. Eat when the body says to eat. Rest when the body says to rest. Exercise and push yourself past the performance level you "think" you can achieve.

The mitochondria release energy. The goal is to enhance mitochondria health so that they have enormous amounts of energy. As your body shifts into the Quantum experience, the mitochondria will be splitting cells into a dimension beyond what you experience now. They will do this through an energetic process wherein the body shifts away from density. You want your body in pristine condition so it can go through the process in the easiest way.

It takes awareness and discipline to read your frequency pattern. Practice listening to what your body is telling you, what it needs to function at a higher spin state. This may seem uncomfortable, even odd, at first.

Your body will show you exactly what you need to do to move into pristine condition to awaken the Quantum Body. Your goal is for your mitochondria to have the power to allow your cells to divide into the Quantum Field of your body.

Why is it so important to listen to the body? You must master the 2nd Light Body, or your thoughts will always be leading, and the body won't have the opportunity to show you that it knows more than you do.

To master the 2nd Light Body, you allow the body to move into expression of Source Intelligence. You allow Consciousness to follow it instead of allowing your body to reflect the Level of Consciousness you are holding.

Allow the activated Codes of DNA Intelligence to take control. Attune to what the body is saying and allow it to show what you need to do. Let the body lead. The body will attune your Consciousness.

In the beginning, the goal is to put the body into optimum health. As you awaken the Quantum Body, your purpose is for Consciousness to meet the Frequency of 963 Hz. held in DMT™. You don't want to leave Consciousness behind.

This is why you use Intuitive Powers to read the Intelligence of DMT until Consciousness merges with the Frequency. (Intuitive Powers are explored in Chapter 8.) You then become that Intelligence. Eventually, Consciousness will become the body.

You begin to consciously connect and attune to the Intelligence held in the Quantum Body. Initially you use reflection to see density in order to shift to a Frequency beyond density. You begin to move past unconscious primal programming and begin to actively use Consciousness to connect to Source Intelligence.

For example, to reverse aging, you co-create with your body, master your biology and override looping cycles held in belief systems. Your body begins to identify as Frequency rather than form.

As you express DNA Intelligence through Frequency, a cell retains the energetic pattern of a cell but not in form; it is no longer dense. The cell no longer identifies as itself within the programmed body and sees itself as Frequency or the Quantum Body. It identifies as an energy system.

3rd Light Body

You will move back and forth between experiencing the Quantum Body and the body as form, a bridge between the 2nd and 3rd Body. The 1st Light Body is the awakening level. In the 2nd Light Body, you see what's there and shift the cell into a new identity. The body remembers it is more than form.

Once the 3rd Light Body awakens, you become very conscious of the Quantum Body and actively participate in the shift from form to Quantum. You are in witness of what's happening biologically. You are aware of the body's shift into energetic form. You participate with the witnessing of it, and there's an agreement that you are ready to move into this experience.

Your agreement allows the shift to begin. You will feel different as your cells hold a higher Frequency. Consciousness merges with the Quantum Body by attuning to DMT™ or activated DNA Intelligence. You experience the cells of your body, organs, tissues and bones in the Quantum Field.

In the 3rd phase, the body will hold form but not as you experience it now. This is "new form." You can see it more as specific software running through a bigger system. Each function of the body will work as Intelligence in communication. In the 3rd Light Body, you create a bridge between form that is connected to space and time and weave into the concept of no space/no time or between space.

In the 3rd Light Body, you begin to identify with the Frequency of the Quantum Body and less with the primal programmed body or density. The cells of the body hold more space, and the spaces between the cells hold more space. The body begins to identify as Frequency, which allows density to shift to Frequency as well. The cells of the body identify as Frequency more than identifying as form.

Your body is already multi-dimensional. You are already the Quantum Body. Because you hold Consciousness in the observation of your own programming, you experience your body as density. As you identify in your Quantum Body, density still exists. But you are in a reality beyond the observation that creates density.

In this phase, you begin to master your biology. You are able to extend telomere length, shift skin cells and see signs of age reversal. The chemical responses of the body shift into Frequency; chemicals no longer exist.

Consciousness merges with the Quantum Body and begins using Intelligence to shift the cells of the body, organs and tissues to hold the Frequency of 963 Hz. It will seem as though a gateway opens that holds space between what you are becoming and what you are holding now.

The Quantum Body holds Source Intelligence and encodes all cells to hold a combination of Codes, 12 to be exact. Twelve Codes are used in different arrangements depending on the density of an organ or tissue.

Your Consciousness, your body on a cellular level, will begin to identify in the Quantum Body. The body becomes a Quantum Frequency because it no longer identifies in form. This indicates that you are moving out of the 2nd Light Body. You are actively turning on your cells to express the Frequency of Source Intelligence. You activate the DNA consciously until your Consciousness completely merges with the

Frequency of DMT™. You actively participate as you move fully into the Quantum Body.

The cells begin to prepare biologically to shift to multidimensional levels of Frequency and release the experience of density. You actively turn on DNA in expression of the Frequency of Source. When you do this over time, the body reaches a Frequency that consciously creates an experience in a Field of no time and no space. DNA is imprinted with DMT™, or Source Intelligence.

When a cell is activated, it begins to transfer Frequency to the surrounding cells. You see this when a healer holds a higher Frequency for someone who is sick; the compromised person meets the higher Frequency and is healed. In this case, the cells transfer a Code through Frequency, shifting a cell to move to the Frequency of the Code itself. Thus, decoding molecular technology!

As the cells transfer DMT™ Codes, the mitochondria build in strength. The mitochondria are the powerhouses of the cell. The body starts producing high amounts of ATP. This allows the cell to shift from the way it holds density/form. Remember, a diet to support making ATP and building the strength of your mitochondria is highly important.

As the mitochondria build in strength, the body is called to do the same. When you build strength when exercising, Lactate is released. Once the body uses up all of its oxygen, it pulls energy from its hydrogen supplies to produce energy for the tissues. Hydrogen knows how to use energy without needing oxygen.

In this phase, Lactate releases a very specific Frequency that attunes with the Frequency of DMT™. DMT, in the 3rd dimension, refers to a chemical that brings in the imprint of your soul when you are born and releases it from the physical body when you die.

DMT™, as referred to here, is a Frequency, not a chemical. You are connecting the Frequency of Lactate with the Frequency of DMT™; they share the same Frequency.

The body begins to release DMT™ in this phase, allowing the body to use Frequency to function. The body becomes its own energy source without the need for energy from outside itself. The cells begin to function within the Frequency of their own energy source. They become Quantum.

When Lactate is released, it begins to activate the Frequency of DMT™ in the Pineal Gland. This signals the DNA to release Source Intelligence, awakening dormant DNA Codes. This Frequency transfers into your Quantum Body. The cell is now an empty vessel that is ready to shift from density to Frequency. In time the cell becomes its own energy center and will no longer have a need for energy from an outside source.

DNA Codes are held in the Frequency of 963 Hz. yet hold 12 Codes of communication. These Codes can be repeated in different combinations. The combinations are held in different ways depending on what tissue is shifting from form to Quantum. For example, the liver would be created in a blend of three DMT™ Codes but in a different pattern than another body part. The liver still exists but in a multidimensional way, holding space for the body to shift from form to Quantum.

This gives the body the ability to still exist but in Frequency. The body shifts from density to Frequency and a gateway for the body to release density has been created. In time, cells stop dividing, dissolve and become Frequency as the mitochondria push through a last force of stored energy held inside them.

Once one cell has been created anew, the body must work to catch up with the shift. The new cell will transfer information from the DMT™ Code to cells still existing in density or form. The process happens slowly. You will feel it occurring. One at a time, a cell will shift and move into multidimensional form. This will happen over time as your body is held in the new cell structure and the empty cells have no function.

You consciously and actively participate in this awakening. Your Consciousness will skyrocket. In Ascension work, there is no bypassing, or it won't happen. You must do every step. Listen to your body and do exactly what it asks.

The body is your Ascension tool. Consciousness alone cannot do it. You must let your body turn on DMT™ Intelligence and actively participate in this Intelligence! This will require awareness and Spiritual Discipline.

Your Quantum System must be connected to Consciousness. This starts in the 1st and 2nd Light Body. By the 3rd Light Body, you must be an active participant in the shift from form to Quantum.

As you embody each level of Consciousness, you expend less energy in the body. You use less oxygen, which allows your body to rebuild itself. Thus, each level is a step in consciously experiencing this evolution. As the body shifts to identifying as Frequency, you expend less energy. As you consciously listen to the Intelligence tell you what the body needs to support this shift, you allow Consciousness to rise at a faster rate.

Everything becomes the Quantum Body. You are the Quantum Body. You are actively aware you are Quantum and that you can retrieve information within the Intelligence stored there. You no longer seek information outside of the Intelligence. You become a human Google system; you **"You-gle"** information as needed.

In the 2nd Light Body, you are actively building the Quantum System by teaching your cells how to shift identity with that awareness. The Frequencies start to activate, and the cells start to move into expression, just like the Sun shines.

All energy responses in the body connect to build and awaken the Quantum Body. Consciously, you are still in the experience of the I AM, observation of yourself, where Consciousness is outside watching the Quantum System activating.

When you move into the 3rd Light Body, Consciousness goes online. Consciousness runs within the Quantum System. This is the bridge between the 3rd and 4th Level of Consciousness. The part of you that identifies outside of the Quantum Body begins to dissipate. You actively participate as the Quantum Body.

Consciousness is experienced beyond form. When you bring your cells online, Consciousness is already aware of what it is to exist beyond the experience of the programmed body.

You may still have the experience of being physical but begin to notice you feel different, that your body is different. You are able to experience and actively participate with your cell division as the Quantum System. The part of you that wants to observe itself to have an experience vanishes.

Practice asking yourself, **"Is my Consciousness witnessing the Quantum System or is it the Quantum System? What would it feel like to actually bring my Consciousness online and become Quantum?"** Fluctuate back and forth between what these feels like. When the chemical response goes away, you will have a new level of mastery over your body. The 3rd Light Body is the Body where you are likely to spend the longest amount of time.

Bridging the 3rd Light Body to the 4th Light Body

Here the imprinted cells are holding DMT™ Codes in multidimensional form without density. You came to this planet to be a part of this pivotal moment. As a Wayshower, an "evolved human," you are the Creator and the Creation of the New Earth.

You are an advanced Soul holding a unique expression of Divine Design. You are a unique experience in the awakening of these Codes. You are a channel that brings through DMT™ Frequencies directly connected in this design. You hold DMT™ Codes that are released. Your brilliance is needed in the world. Many of you have been afraid to release the need to stay small and your repetition of old stories and belief systems. It is time to become your NEXT. To show yourself and your gifts to the world.

For far too long as an Evolved Human, you have hidden behind your programming, feeling trapped in a wheel of repeated behavior for which you judge and shame yourself. You are an advanced being stuck in an old paradigm of healing and change.

What if you remembered that you are already 100% Source Intelligence and that all you have to do is self-discover in your highest potential? Isn't it time to step into your power and discover who you are beyond your programming?

This cannot be done by focusing on where you have repeatedly looked. Your ego mind wants you to believe that you need to do more before you can be happy, abundant or successful. This is not true. You are called to see yourself as whole, as perfect in this now moment.

You already have the highest level of Source Intelligence within you. It cannot awaken when you focus on needing to be fixed. You can bring through information, insights and Quantum Technology in this moment just by being you.

What would life be like if you chose to know this instead of holding yourself in fear and judgment? You are here to assist in activating Higher Consciousness so needed in the World. You hold the very magic your heart desires. Are you ready to step into your brilliance? Are you ready to claim yourself to be the Quantum Human? To let go of programmed instructions for how to manifest, become more spiritual or enlightened?

The old way of achieving your highest potential is far outdated. Your growth as an advanced being allows you to access Higher Intelligence immediately. You are a transmitter of Source Intelligence and are here to awaken the Quantum Body. You are ready to awaken DMT™ Codes and experience higher Frequencies to create change.

As you connect to your Quantum Self, you will remember who you are in your highest potential. In this moment, commit to focusing on who you are in this magical space. Become the spiritual alchemist you are here to be.

4th Light Body

In this body, you connect to Frequency without space or beyond connection to space. You turn on an expression of self-empowerment. You recognize that it's through your choices, Spiritual Discipline and bridging techniques that you create higher spin states in the body.

You consciously attune to higher Frequencies to experience bigger shifts or changes in your body. Your body and Consciousness identify as Frequency. The imprinted cells hold the Frequency of DMT™ in multidimensional form.

Your cells now express Frequency without identifying as form or density. This allows the body to function perfectly without using energy from outside itself. It becomes its own energy source as Source Intelligence.

The body becomes a Quantum System or Technology. The organs, breath, blood and nervous system move completely online and no longer exist in the first 3 Levels or the programmed body. Consciousness is now held in the Quantum System and is fully online.

Mind and matter are related in the 4th Light Body as the mind becomes Quantum. The body's responses to its environment shift completely as the body becomes a vibrational pattern beyond the first 3 Bodies.

The nervous system dissolves, leaving an imprinted pattern that moves into the Quantum System of Intelligence. This creates a boost in energy the Quantum Body needs to fully function as its own sustained energy source. If done consciously, the mind fully moves into this energy and becomes the Intelligence held in the Quantum Body without reflection. This is the 5th Level of Consciousness.

Particles and energy are connected through electrons in the 4th Body. You master the existence of the field that was once perceived as your environment. The 4th and 5th Bodies begin to work together with your participation in the creation of the 5th Light Body until you become it. The 5th Body is 100% Human Potential. The Advanced Human!

Right now, you're likely experiencing the field as something around you or outside of you. Quantum Physics is based on the reality that the mind has to be present, the observer, in order to create reality. This is because the observer itself is creating this reality.

In the 4th Body, there is nothing that exists outside of the Intelligence of you as a Quantum Body or System. Observation is a reflection of Consciousness within the Field. You can "Break Quantum Physics."

The mind/Consciousness/self merges with the Intelligence that is the Quantum Field, or Source Intelligence, without the need for reflection or observation. The Quantum Field shifts to expression of the Intelligence held in Self as the very Intelligence of what once was observed as the field. This disintegrates the field as it is now and opens up a reality that has not yet been discovered.

5th Light Body

In this body, you exist without holding space or the connection to space. You are able to hold an expression without reflection. You exist without existing. As a Quantum Body or Frequency of Intelligence, Consciousness shifts into the Intelligence running the Technology of the body itself.

You become Source Intelligence in the expression of energy or waves that exist without reflection. You are the Creator and the Creation at the same time as the Advanced Body or Human. You hold no space and no time because you are no longer in observation or reflection.

At first, you experience this consciously until Consciousness completely merges as the Intelligence. The Quantum Field no longer exists because no observation of an intelligence in observation exists. At this moment the 5th Light Body fully activates. You become Source Intelligence, the 5th Level of Consciousness.

Notes

Notes

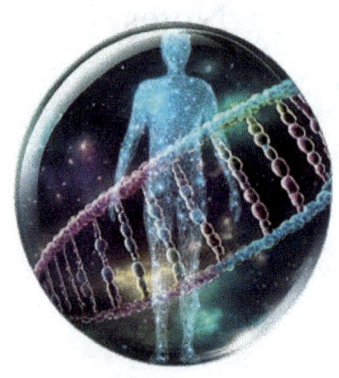

Chapter 5: The Evolution Technology: Learning The Symbols Of Lu, Sca, 33

"The keys to life are the Pyramids of Light that live inside of everything. Evolution can be programmed to a higher spin state at any time. You can raise up to a higher vibration and hold this vibration through Consciousness held in the Frequency of the Spin State. Pyramid energy is a central form of all evolution. The Hydrogen Atom controls the spin, the orientation of everything in our Universe, shifting from reflection to expression. The Pyramid is the gateway of Consciousness and fuses space, time and matter to no space and no time. The Pyramid on top of a Pyramid is a vehicle of Ascension." ~Unknown

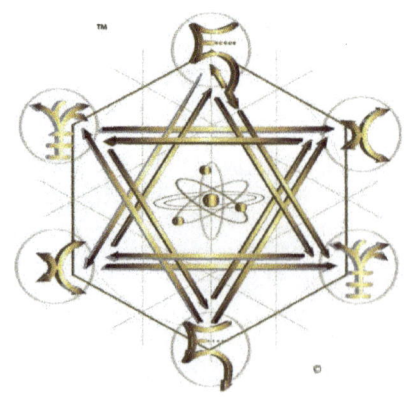

Jewels Story:

"The symbols of the Evolution Technology have been with me most my life. I was five years old when they first came to me. I used them to soothe myself, especially at night before going to bed. I'd see them floating around me and with my mind I'd bring them into my mind's eye. As they entered my brain, I would immediately feel relaxed. By the time the 33 entered my mind, I would drift off into sleep.

As I grew, they would come in and out of my life. It wasn't until 2020 that I started sharing them with others as they hold the Scalar Frequency Technology of the Evolution Symbol. From here, others began to attune to their power, using them as a delivery system that shifts the cells, energy patterns and reality from observation of the Field to expression of Source Intelligence. In this chapter you will learn to use the Lu, Sca and 33 to shift your cells to higher spin states and awaken DMT™."

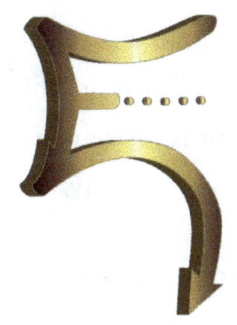

Lu: Luminous, the 1st Evolution Symbol, dissolves all frequencies held in the Matrix or programmed body, creating no time and no space or Zero Point. The **Lu** neutralizes anything that has taken on programming or form, brings thoughts to a still point and clears static energy in your body or reality. Bring the Symbol into the static and allow it to spin. If using the **Lu** for something physical, bring the Symbol directly into the cells of that area. See the **Lu** spinning inside your cells. Notice the shift.

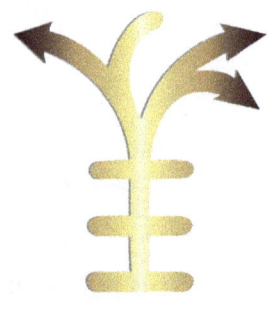
Sca: Scalar, the 2nd Symbol in Evolution Technology, is used to bring through the 7 Elements. (The 7 Elements are taught in the next chapter.) **Sca** allows Consciousness to be held in no time and no space. After **Lu** creates Zero Point, **Sca** is activated and DMT™ releases. **Sca** releases Intelligence by turning on dormant DNA Codes. **Sca** is key to unlocking DMT™ Frequencies.

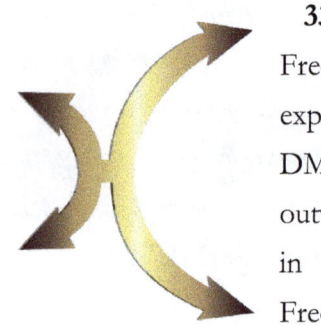
33: The 3rd Evolution Symbol moves the Frequency of activated DNA Codes into expression of Pure Source Intelligence or DMT™. The **33** pushes the Frequency of Source outward from the cell. This allows the cells to stay in expression, beyond observation. As the Frequency of DMT™ expresses, the first 3 Levels of the body begin to dissolve and bypass the programming that holds the DNA in observation of its environment. When in the expression of DMT™ Intelligence, the looping system is broken and you exist in an Intelligence beyond the programmed body or reality.

This diagram shows how the Evolution Technology holds the Foundation of the Quantum Body. You will now learn the next 2 Pyramids, the 7 Elements and the God Sphere.

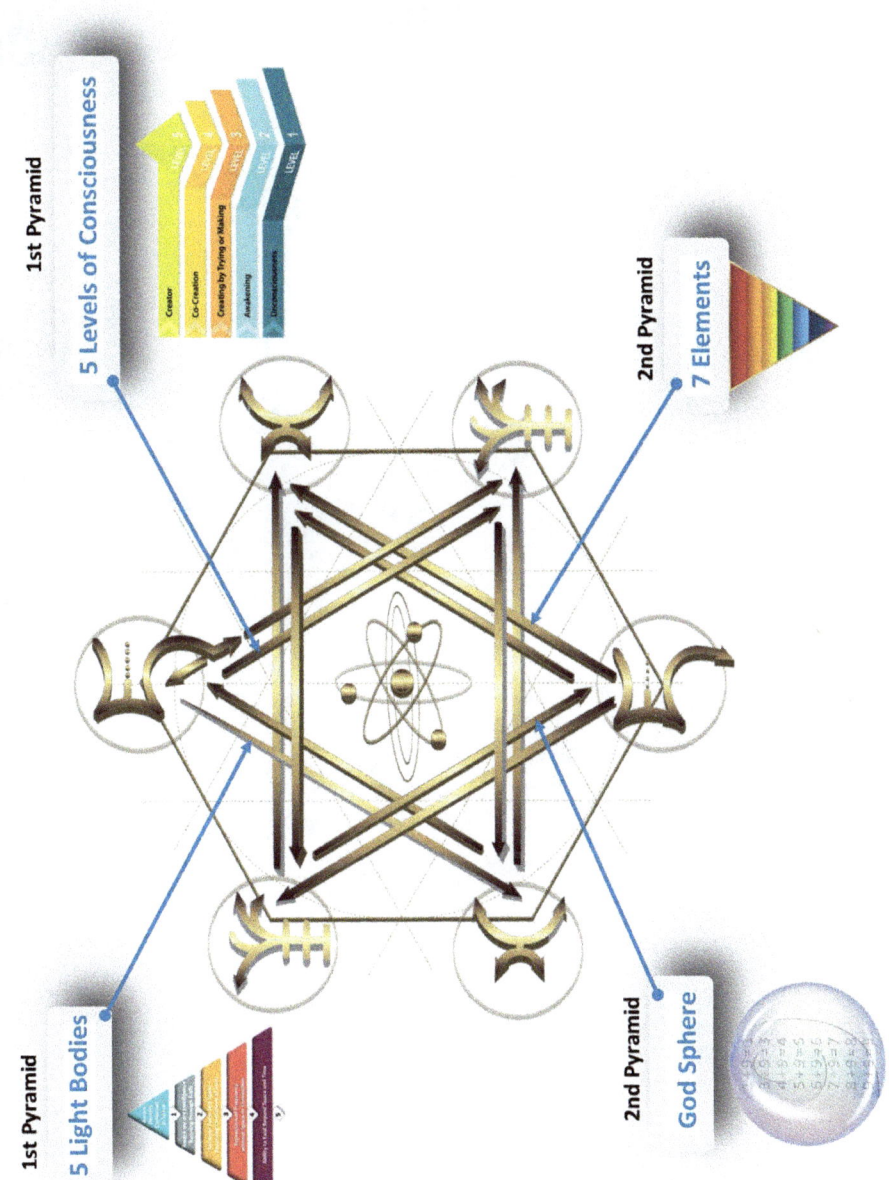

Notes

Notes

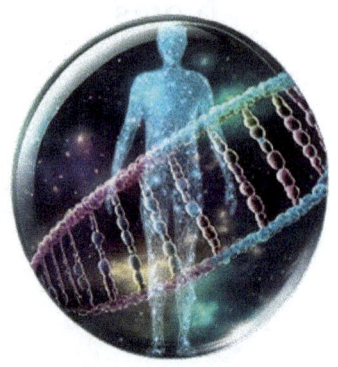

Chapter 6: The 7 Elements

The 2nd Pyramid of Evolution Technology

The 2nd Pyramid of the Evolution Symbol holds tools of awareness within a programmed state. The Technologies of the two Pyramids are the 7 Elements and the God Sphere. If the word "God" is uncomfortable in any way, replace it with a word you prefer. The word God is used because it illustrates how to master That perceived as God and demonstrates how to move beyond identifying not only in the words, but identity all together.

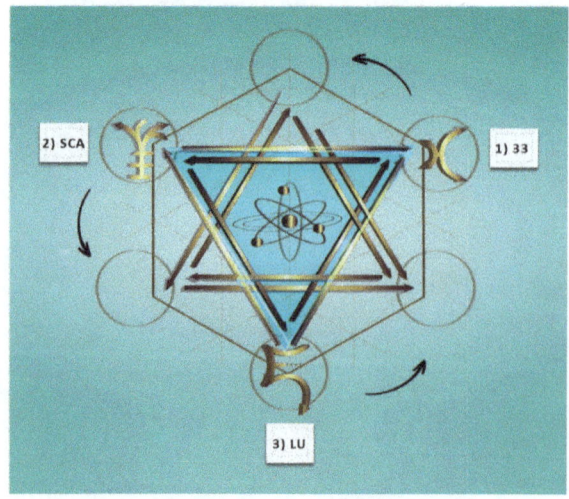

As you awaken the Quantum Body, you master the States of Consciousness. First, you become aware of the Level in which you are existing. There are 7 States you will use to move beyond the programmed mind and body.

Each State of Consciousness is connected to a multidimensional Element that absorbs into the mind and body and brings the cells into a higher spin state. As you work with the Elements, be aware that these cannot be mastered through intellect. They must be absorbed as a state of being beyond what can be understood by the mind.

Imagine an Element as something that feeds the cells nutrition to be healthy and strong. The 7 Elements feed the Quantum Body and strengthen an organic system beyond programming held in the first 3 Levels of the body.

Transformation of the 7 Elements:

The 7 Elements work together in 5 States of Consciousness. Each is absorbed through a scalar light wave that transcends the programmed mind and body.

As light waves enter the brain, you begin to absorb them. Your brain changes as Light merges with the cells, neurotransmitters and the overall programmed mind. The Light cannot be penetrated, only absorbed. You absorb the Light of the 7 Elements to master the Ascended Mind.

When the mind is fully resonating with the Frequency or Intelligence of each Element, you notice a shift in Consciousness. There is more space between the chatter in your mind. Your mind becomes a transmitter to attune to Source or DMT™ Intelligence. You are not your mind, and your mind is not separate from Source.

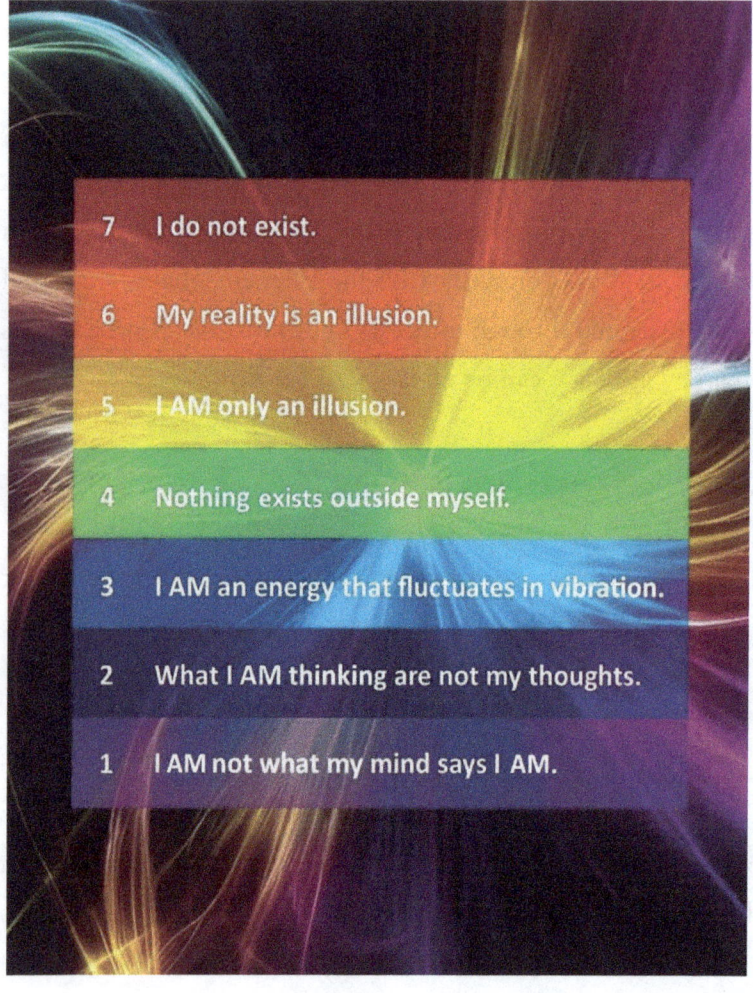

The 7 Elements: https://becomingbioquantum.com/7Elements

You are breaking infinity so that karma, time and space stop repeating. Time stays the same because there is no time. Karma, or cause and effect, cannot exist when in expression of Source Intelligence. Your ego does not exist when Consciousness meets Source Intelligence. You are just Intelligence without reflection because reflection is not needed.

The 7 Elements are a pathway to manifest deeper integration into the mind through States of Consciousness. Avoid trying to understand this. Rather, ask for an awareness of a State of Consciousness and then observe awareness come forth.

The 7 Elements:

>**1st Element:** I AM Not My Mind. I AM Not What My Mind Says I AM.
>**2nd Element:** I AM Not My Thoughts. What I AM Thinking Are Not My Thoughts.
>**3rd Element:** I AM Not My Body. I AM Energy That Fluctuates In Vibration.
>**4th Element:** Nothing Exists Outside Myself.
>**5th Element:** I AM Only An Illusion.
>**6th Element:** My Reality Is An Illusion.
>**7th Element:** I Do Not Exist.

The 1st Element: Element of the Violet Ray: "I AM Not My Mind."

What keeps you from experiencing Source or Universal Intelligence is the observation of the Matrix or programmed reality. The 1st Element, **"I AM Not My Mind,"** will support your connection with Source. You are not your mind, and your mind is not separate from the Universe. What keeps you from becoming the identity you wish to be, or to evolve beyond identity altogether, is a *switch* inside your mind that needs to be mastered. The 1st Element will support this.

See your mind as separate from you and not your identity. View it as a machine that has been programmed through experiences, repeated thought patterns and by downloads absorbed from others.

It is time to move past why you are the way you are, why you are programmed this way. See your mind as a machine that you have the ability to reprogram. To reprogram, you first have to see what is there and clear out what you no longer want in order to make room for the new. You basically choose to redecorate your mind, very much like you would do your home.

As the Violet Scalar Light Wave awakens the brain, it works with the Pituitary Gland, reprogramming the chemical responses in the body. This master gland is an intricate system in itself.

Once you move beyond the programmed body, the Pituitary Gland begins to work with the Pineal Gland by releasing Frequencies holding Source Intelligence. You become able to respond to your environment beyond primal programming, beyond what you perceive as reality. As the Pituitary and Pineal Glands reprogram and work together, DMT™ Codes awaken. The DNA begins to express Frequencies beyond programming.

As you absorb the 1st Element, and practice the state of Consciousness, **"I Am Not My Mind,"** your DNA ceases to reproduce lower frequency gene codes. This is the beginning of dissolving genetic dysfunction. This is the evolution of the New Human and of mankind. Your cells transform to become Divinely perfect.

The 1st Element opens a doorway to choice and empowerment and makes you aware that your past is just a story stored in the brain and then reflected into the reality you are experiencing. The only way you create a new reality, or reprogram the cells to higher levels of Intelligence, is by becoming aware that you are not your mind.

You are not the story held in your mind, and you have the ability to change everything! Every time you think you are stuck, tired and not happy with what you are experiencing, interrupt the thought pattern by bringing attention to the thoughts you are having. Think about what you desire to experience.

What I AM statement or higher Frequency reality do you wish to create? Hold the new thought in your mind's eye and see it rewire your brain. Really watch it happen. Then ask yourself, *"Who am I when I am in the Frequency of this new thought?"*

Start thinking in this new identity. *"What am I feeling, experiencing? How do I act, speak, relate to the people around me?"* It's a practice to rewire the brain to higher Frequency realities. You are not your brain. You are the master of the machine that is your brain! How do you want to wire it?

You will want to resist and go back into thoughts of lack, suffering or old patterns. You will be tempted to "figure out your problems" so that you feel safe. These moments offer an opportunity to rewire to your new identity just by observing yourself and not repeating old patterns.

In these moments say, **"I am creating a reality of freedom from my mind. I am the master of my mind, and I choose to experience _____ right now."** Now count backward from 10 to 1 and interrupt your pattern by doing five jumping jacks, singing a song, going for a walk or anything that changes up your energy. Listen to a podcast or music that is inspiring. Refocus and do something that raises your frequency. It may feel like nothing is happening. Trust and know you are rewiring and creating a new reality.

Every time you question why you are the way you are, decide who it is you want to be. Create an image that holds the reality of your desires and practice becoming that. This is referred to as creating an Avatar. As the cells hold the new identity with an "I AM" statement, it gives the conscious mind something to become.

I AM Statements:
https://becomingbioquantum.com/IAmStatements
Exercise: Creating an Avatar:

Create a powerful I AM statement that expresses who you wish to become. Feel the Frequency of your new identity and take the time to develop your new persona.

For example, in creating the Avatar, **"I AM Brave,"** consider how your life would be different and ask yourself the following questions:

> *Who am I if I AM brave?*
> *How do I go through my day if I AM brave?*
> *What are my thoughts and feelings if I AM brave?*
> *What do I look like if I AM brave?*
> *What do I wear if I AM brave?*
> *How do I speak to myself and others if I AM brave?*
> *In what other ways will my life shift if I AM brave?*

Allow yourself to attune to this new version of you. Allow the person you are now to merge into your Avatar. Feel into the Frequency and fully embrace your new identity. Have fun playing! Become the master of your destiny!

Even if you think you know why you are the way you are, it doesn't change your future. It just gives you a story to explain "why" you are a victim. You are only a victim of you. You recreate the story or your experiences over and over and may look for something or someone to blame. There is no one to blame! You can choose to create a new reality.

Ask Universal Intelligence to support you in seeing the beliefs, programs and thoughts that repeat inside your brain so that you can rewire to higher Frequency thoughts you have not experienced before. Your brain is not you.

The brain is a machine you, as a master, can use to create whatever reality you put your focus on. Start to observe what thoughts you are programming into your mind. Are they holding the reality you want to create? If not, you have a choice to design something different. This is the 2nd Level of Consciousness.
You are AWARE!

Observe and repeat the method above to start rewiring your mind to hold your desired reality. Even better, ask Source Intelligence to show you your NEXT. Can you let go of trying to make it happen and let information come in from beyond your programming? Remind yourself, **"I AM the Creator of my life. I AM capable of reprogramming my reality to the highest potential for me right now. I remain curious and explore my future."**

Simply absorb the 1st Element and witness with the part of you that is observing the mind itself. This Element is awakening Consciousness in the Quantum Body. Explore or be curious about who you are beyond the programming of your mind.

Meditation of the Violet Light:

Place your hands on your heart and start to breathe up and down the channel along your spine, running through the top of your head and down out your root chakra. Breathe in as the energy moves up; breathe out as the energy moves down.

Start to relax and let go of any thoughts or worries as the gateway within this channel expands out from your body. The energy expands out, filling your body with the Light of Source. It expands out even further as it fills your aura with a beautiful golden Light. You feel safe and protected in this Light.

With your hands on your heart, tone the sound "Eeeeeee." With this sound you are calling in the 7 Scalar Lights of the Prism that holds the 7 Elements. Feel the vibration of this tone in your heart. Again, tone the sound "Eeeeeee." Call in the 7 Rays of the Prism in the Eye of Source. Feel the vibration of this sound in your heart. Once again, tone the sound "Eeeeeee." Feel your heart open and allow the 7 Rays to enter the Chambers of your heart.

Before you is a beautiful Pyramid. The Light of the Ascended Sun shines down through the Pyramid and penetrates the 7 Rays of Light even further into your heart. The Light Rays shimmer with an elegance beyond words. Allow your heart to absorb the Light; let it fill your body and your aura. The Rays of Light merge with the golden Light of Source. You feel the Light enter your cells and molecules, raising your vibration. Relax into the Frequency of the Light Rays.

You feel a Presence beside you. The Ascended Body of your Higher Self asks for permission to enter your physical body and brings you on a journey through the Light Rays so that you may absorb the 7 Elements. You feel the love of your Higher Self and look forward to the journey. As you embrace the Light of your Higher Self, you become One.

In this new state of being, as One with your Higher Self, you begin to float down a hallway within your heart. You see the door of the first Chamber. It holds the Violet Light. Within the Violet Light is the 1st Element: **"I AM Not What My Mind Says I AM."**

Opening the big heavy door, you step into the Chamber of the Violet Light. In front of you, there is a transmitter connected to a copper Pyramid crown. You sit in a comfortable chair and allow the guides of this room to fit the Pyramid onto your head. You shut your eyes as the electric pulses of the Violet Light enter your mind and fill your head with the Frequency needed to activate the dormant parts of your brain. Your mind relaxes and lets go of the need to control. The lower mind loses energy as the Violet Light activates the higher brain, bringing the mind into Universal Consciousness. Feel the Violet Light balancing the mind and letting go of low vibration programming.

You now have access to the Frequencies needed to continue on your journey. Expand out into the cosmos and absorb the knowledge of the stars. Let go of any thoughts and become the stars. Use the machine of the mind to connect to the template of the Universe. Your higher mind becomes an intricate system of Frequencies that bring you further into the Violet Light.

The 2nd Element: Element of the Indigo Ray: "What I Think Are Not My Thoughts."

The color of the second Ascended Scalar Light Wave is Indigo. The 1st and 2nd Elements teach you to be the observer of your thoughts. When you check in with yourself and ask, **"What am I thinking?"** you become the observer and realize that you have a choice between being the programmer or the program. When you are in the program, you are in the 1st Level of Consciousness, the primal body.

Practice being the observer and the Creator at the same time. Watch your thoughts as you do repetitive chores such as doing dishes or brushing your teeth. Ask yourself, **"Is it important for me to be thinking what I'm thinking?"** If it is not, use these times to practice Mindfulness. Become aware of your thoughts and then bring your attention back to the task at hand. Make this your daily practice.

The Quantum Body is the part of you that is watching yourself think your thoughts. Many thoughts you experience are not your thoughts. Thoughts are energy. The mind creates thought when picking up an energetic vibration floating around your environment. Remember that the first environment of your Consciousness is your body.

There are different frequencies of thoughts that can alter your moods and how you create your reality. Thoughts are energies that are tuned into, just like a radio picking up a signal. The frequency at which you are vibrating determines the station of thoughts you will pick up. No matter what station you tune into, these are still not your thoughts. The mind is a transmitter of energy that sends and receives messages connected to programming. The higher your frequency, the higher the vibration of thoughts you will tune into. Look at thoughts as information and decide whether you agree with them.

Thoughts can be from your outer or inner environment. The inner environment, your mind and body, holds past frequency patterns or programs you pick up as you move through life. Most are programmed between the ages of one to seven years. These programs can be seen as energy patterns that were passed from person to person without Consciousness. They are not to be judged, analyzed, nor to create stories from, though that is what you unconsciously do. *This is how you become who you are in this moment.*

Everyone around you has thoughts. These thoughts are dispersed into a matrix of energy which becomes absorbed into the Matrix or an energy field holding the vibrations of thought. The Matrix holds even thoughts that you think have never been discovered. There are no new thought patterns, only new levels of becoming conscious of Source Intelligence. You enter different vibrational frequencies where thoughts and information enter through electric responses of your body's electrons and are registered in repeated patterns in the brain.

All thoughts come from a Field or Frequency grid holding Source Intelligence, which holds the Consciousness of every energy being in existence. How you experience this Intelligence is dependent on your level of Consciousness. There are three thought forms you will be working with:

- *Conscious Thought*
- *Unconscious Thought*
- *Super-conscious Thought*

Conscious Thought:

Conscious thoughts are the part of the mind that houses the ego and are to be challenged in order for you to awaken the Quantum Body. They have a purpose: your grocery list, directions, or remembering where you put your keys. These thoughts are stored in the mind and are used to recall information. Most thoughts you tune into have no purpose and keep you stuck in social or ego consciousness.

Have you ever had something arise and you go over it hundreds of times trying to find a solution but never do? Do you find yourself repeating the same story or thought, thinking you can control the outcome? Such thoughts are of a low vibration, are abundant in the programmed body and create attachments in anyone that resonates with them.

Thoughts repeated become programs. Programs are thoughts agreed upon consciously or unconsciously. When seen with the mind's eye, these thoughts appear as deep ruts in the brain that have very low pulses of energy. When you have experiences that trigger these thoughts, you have a similar response.

Have you ever noticed you have the same feeling over and over to different experiences that cause you stress? This is a programmed response to a thought or belief system deep in the Unconscious Mind.

Programs create chemical reactions in the body and keep you stuck in low vibrations. It all starts with a thought you agreed to, a thought that was never yours to begin with. Some examples of low vibrational thoughts or social consciousness are:

I will never make it in life because I am not smart enough.
I have to work hard in order to survive.
How I dress and what I own shows my social status.
I dress to impress so I will not be judged.
My children are a reflection of how good a parent I am.
My parents have bad genes, so I will too.
Religion is the way to salvation.
Aging is inevitable.
If I play small, I will not be seen.
If I am not seen, I will not be humiliated if I fail.
If I don't agree with others, I will be alone.
Being mainstream and not questioning my life keeps me safe.

These and other low-frequency thoughts keep you stuck in a low vibration. Become aware that you are not your thoughts. They are a frequency of an energy vibrating in the station you are resonating in.

Unconscious Thought:

Unconscious thoughts are thoughts that live in the Subconscious Mind. They are always whispering in the background without your knowledge. These are programs that control you without you even knowing it. Unconscious thoughts tell you who you are and are programmed with the instinct to survive. Unconscious thoughts are powerful. They can trap you in a very low state of consciousness.

These programs hold energy connected to:

Need to control others or yourself to feel safe
Need to be the best or hide your power

> *Manipulation*
> *Judgment*
> *Fear of death*
> *Survival at all costs*
> *Fear of suffering*
> *Feeling responsible for those you love*
> *Feeling not good enough*
> *If they know who I am, they will find out I am not important.*
> *I am not smart or capable.*
> *I can't handle my life.*
> *I am unworthy.*
> *I am unlovable.*
> **...And many other programs of *duality*.**

These are the underlying programs you live by every day, keeping you unconscious.

To **"awaken,"** bring these programs into the conscious mind by discovering they are not real. They are just an illusion that makes you feel safe. They represent the primal body connected to the 1st Level of Consciousness, the Unconscious Mind.

Unconscious thoughts are connected to chemical responses in the brain. When they start to play, unaware the thoughts are there, you trigger with fear, anxiety and panic. This response offers the Conscious Mind the chance to come online. In order to feel safe or in control, the Conscious Mind creates a story about the feelings that have been triggered. The story is a low vibrational thought that is not who you are and most likely is not true.

Superconscious Thoughts:

Superconscious thoughts assist you in overcoming unconscious and conscious thoughts. The Superconscious is the part of the mind that resonates at a Frequency that can bring you into higher states of Consciousness. Thoughts come into challenge programs that play automatically, control you and keep you stuck. This part of the mind is the Observer. This is the voice you hear when you stop the mind chatter and start asking questions such as, **"Is this a necessary thought?"**

The Superconscious Mind is able to rise above thoughts that vibrate in low vibrations and offer the opportunity to choose differently. At first, it can be difficult to hear the Superconscious. But the more you listen, the easier it becomes. Programming of social consciousness becomes a whisper, and you become the master of your mind. You are on your way to knowing, **"I AM Not My Thoughts. I AM Not My Mind."**

Here are some examples of thoughts of the Superconscious:

> *Am I acting out my fears?*
> *Do I need to feel afraid in this situation?*
> *Am I manipulating the outcome to be in control?*
> *What is really going on?*
> *What do I need to look at so I can see beyond the illusion of this experience?*
> *Why do I feel I need to act as though I am more or less than I am? Do I see that I exaggerate or dumb it down in order to feel important, safe or to create connection?*
> *Do I need to work on just telling the truth and knowing that it is enough?*

Do I see myself wanting to control this situation in order to feel safe? I can see this is a program that plays out when I fear suffering. Am I safe right now? Am I reacting appropriately?
Am I really in danger or is this just my need to control?
I am getting angry because others are not acting the way I think they should. What program am I playing out?
Do I feel unlovable? Unimportant?

Observe how you are reacting and what programs are playing out. Thoughts of the Superconscious Mind detach you from thoughts, keeping you stuck in social consciousness or past programs and give you awareness to break the cycle. We call this ***"Breaking the Brain Loop."*** *You move into the 2nd Level of Consciousness, the Awakening Level or where you become aware.* Become the Observer of the mind and thoughts. Use the thoughts of the Superconscious Mind to awaken.

Exercise:

Start challenging your thoughts as if they were advice from a friend with whom you love to debate. **"Do I need to be thinking this? What am I trying to accomplish? Do I need to feel in control? Safe? Justified? Is this true for me? Do I like the way this thought makes me feel? How long have I had this thought? Is there a feeling within this thought that I need to go deeper into and explore? What unconscious thought is controlling me?"**

Don't stop challenging a thought until you can name it for what it is. Become aware of the pattern and the programs behind it. Step into Quantum Consciousness. When you are aware of the thought patterns that keep you stuck, *you have a choice*. You can choose to agree or not. You take back your power with awareness.

Meditation of the Indigo Ray:

You have mastered the Violet Ray and are ready to move into the next Chamber of your heart. You feel the shift in your mind and Consciousness. The guides of the Violet Chamber hug you goodbye while asking that the Pyramid crown remain on your head throughout the journey.

You start to walk down the hall to the Chamber of the Indigo Ray. Each step you take brings you into a deep state of relaxation. Your breath slows. Your thoughts and worries float away. You feel safe and protected within the Chambers of your heart. Ahead, you notice a soft glow coming from under the door of the Indigo Chamber. You feel an excitement stir within you as you open the door. The light is coming from a candle burning on an old antique table with an elegant soft chair next to it. The light of the candle radiates an Indigo flame that mesmerizes you. The guides of this room are different but emanate the same love.

You sit in the chair and notice a pen and paper in front of you. The guides explain that the pen holds words of Truth and can only write that Truth. They tell you the Truth comes from a transcribed Intelligence in your DNA and writing with this pen will teach you to resonate with the Thoughts of Source.

One of the guides hands you a beautiful clear quartz crystal. You hold the crystal in your hands, and it begins to shine an Indigo Ray of Light that turns into a Pyramid just as it enters your 3rd Eye. The Pyramid on top of a Pyramid creates a heightened state of intuition.

This Pyramid structure within the brain brings the Pituitary Gland into the Pineal Gland and aligns the mind to Universal Truth. The Indigo Ray raises the vibration of your mind and creates a grid for the words of Source to be stored within you. The outline of the grid begins to glow as the synapse responses and neurotransmitters of the brain, storing fight or flight responses, gently dissipate and lose control over you.

The Indigo Light holds the vibration of thoughts held in the DNA or DMT™ Frequencies. Experience these codes download into your Conscious Mind now. You are here to experience your innate being. As you sit with the Indigo Ray, the 2nd Element, **"I AM Not My Thoughts,"** absorbs into your being.

Your thoughts merge with DMT™ Frequencies and all thoughts connected to your programming fade away, losing their power over you. Pick up the pen and begin to write. Stay in the Light of the Indigo Ray as the words emerge onto the paper before you. Without judgment or fear, connect to Source Consciousness through the 2nd Element. You are changing brain pathways that hold low states of consciousness and reconnecting to Source Intelligence through the DMT™ Codes. Feel at peace as you connect to Universal Truth.

The 3rd Element: Element of the Blue Ray: "I Am Energy that Fluctuates in Vibration."

The 3rd Scalar Light Wave is blue and holds the 3rd Element. Sit with yourself and allow the energy of your body to come to your attention. What do you feel? Sit with it even longer. Now, what do you feel? Yes, you are energy. You are a dense form of energy in a solid form, with a mind and thoughts that tell you who you are and what you see because those that came before you agreed to this reality. When a thought is agreed to by the masses, it becomes social consciousness or programmed reality. This state of Consciousness is why you believe you are your body.

The more you believe you are a body, the denser your body becomes and the more you stay in the programming or experience of the first 3 Levels of the body. The vibration of your thoughts creates the environment you live in, your body. As you challenge your thoughts and clear the programming of the first 3 Bodies, you vibrate at a higher Frequency.

Higher Frequencies vibrate with the particles in your body because you are the energy of these particles. Low vibrational thoughts move very slowly; their energies cluster together and create a dense mass that attracts slow-vibrating particles that make you feel solid.

You are not a victim of the frequency at which you are vibrating. Thus, other people, your environment and your experiences do not have control over how you choose to experience your environment. You create your reality through choice, the 2nd Level of Consciousness.

You have a **Home Frequency** wherein you naturally vibrate. Your Home Frequency tends to be high. Notice when you lower your frequency to create connection with another. You always have a choice. When you recognize that you are lowering your frequency, observe what's happening, what thoughts you are having. Explore what you absorbed from outside yourself or what you unconsciously connected to.

When around others, it is natural for your body to want to resonate with your environment. If you are conscious, you can choose to hold your Home Frequency regardless of what is occurring outside of you. Your Frequency can upgrade the frequencies of those around you. With your conscious intent, you can invite others to hold a higher Frequency.

Exercise:

Sit with yourself and allow the energy of your body to come to your attention. What do you feel? Sit with it even longer. Now, what do you feel? Take a few moments and bring your attention to your High Heart. This is a gateway to the Quantum Body and holds your Home Frequency.

Bring your Super Conscious Mind into this space, just above your physical heart. Ask to feel your Home Frequency. Sit for a moment and notice if something awakens within you. Do you feel a shift? Continue practicing this exercise until you become aware of how your Home Frequency feels and what it doesn't feel like. This is a tool that will benefit you as you become more sensitive to frequency or energy.

You are energy. You experience this energy in the reflection of your Consciousness as a dense form of energy or solid form. You observe yourself with the programmed mind and thoughts that tell you who you are and what you see because those that came before you agreed to this reality. Is it true?

Exploring your reality through the Super Conscious Mind will bring you to a higher Frequency and change how you experience your cellular structure. You are so much more than your programmed body and mind. You have thoughts but your true being is the energy in between the thoughts.

The Void, or Source Intelligence, is the place of stillness that is your innate being. The Frequency held here contains the essence of the Soul. You are only energy, and you are always moving. Your thoughts will determine the frequency at which your energy vibrates. The next time you feel uncomfortable, recognize it for what it is; it is energy vibrating at a lower frequency.

Your body is made of conscious electrons and energy within a cellular structure. As you move into higher states of Consciousness, the space within your cellular structure becomes wider, allowing more space to be held. As more space is held between density or programming, your Frequency rises.

This vibration is the vehicle that will assist you in creating higher Frequency realities and to reprogram your cells as the Quantum Body awakens. You will meet a vibration your mind cannot understand in its current frequency.

It may seem hard to imagine yourself as energy because your mind is attached to experiencing you as solid form or the programmed body. You are not your body; you are energy. Allow the Elements of Light to absorb into your body. To know you are energy, you must let go of the mind and the need to understand or have evidence. You are invited to exist in a space beyond form or programmed reality. Rest in the space within yourself and know that the energy of your being is moving into a vibration beyond your understanding.

Meditation of the Blue Ray

Feeling connected to Source, you know the Chamber of the Indigo Element is always here for you to return to. The pen that writes the words of Source will be there for you to use when you feel the need for Guidance. Looking around, you are ready to move into the next Chamber of your heart. The guides of the Indigo room kiss your cheek and send you down the hallway to the door of the Blue Element.

The entry is an old ancient castle door. It is beautifully carved with elegant roses around the curved archway. You hear humming from under the door and wonder what it could be coming from. You push open the door and see the guides of the Blue Chamber. They are softly humming in a voice that seems beyond human. They see you enter and fill with excitement as they glide over to you after anxiously awaiting your arrival.

You feel peace and enthusiasm in their presence. Your guides bring you over to a window in the center of a wall laced in blue morning glories. The smell of the soft flowers fills the room, welcoming the Element of the Blue Light into your body. You feel the Element absorbing through your skin, giving you an energy that heightens all of your senses.

As your vibration rises, you notice you are only particles of energy. You look at your body and see it glowing as a brilliant golden light. You feel fluid and light as air as you move. As you reach the window, you have the feeling you could fly. And you do! You lift right off the ground and slip through the window.

One of the guides leads you to review different parts of your life. You see yourself as a child in school being teased by an older child. As you retrace this memory, you feel your body changing and becoming heavy. The guide takes your hand and shares that when you feel pain, your Light loses its ability to shine, and you become dense. You understand that you are energy and that reliving this experience lowered your vibration. You are exhilarated to understand you are truly energy and you desire to experience more.

The guide flies with you over a small town in the country. You see fields of flowers that seem to go on forever. Filled with the lovely sight of these flowers, your body expands into pure Light. You look down, expecting you will no longer be there. But it is you that has changed. You see the particles within you dancing around in the glory of your Light.

Bliss overtakes you and you feel that you could expand and become "all that is." The guide explains that you're vibrating in the Frequency of Love. Your body fully absorbs the Element of the Blue Ray. Your guide takes you back to the Blue Light Chamber and you float gently back onto the stone floor of this glorious room.

You have a deep understanding of **"I AM Energy That Fluctuates in Vibration."** What an amazing Element! The knowledge you received through this experience gives you a new way of looking at life. You are only energy. You affect one another.

The guides fill you with the Blue Light so that you can share this love with all you encounter. You ask yourself, **"What vibration do I wish to vibrate at? What keeps me in a lower vibration? My thoughts! But my thoughts are not mine, so the choice to raise in vibration is always there. I am not a victim of my life. I am a victim of my** thoughts. I choose to no longer be a victim of my thoughts. I am free! I choose to live in the vibration of DMT™, 963 Hz."

The 4th Element: Element of the Green Ray: "Nothing Exists Outside Myself."

The 4th Element is the Green Scalar Light Wave. Imagine you hold everything in the Universe and beyond inside of you. The mountains, the valleys, the stars and planets are all inside your Consciousness and are being reflected into what you perceive to be your reality.

Nothing exists outside of yourself. Everything that has a vibration or Frequency is inside of you supporting your experience of the Quantum Body or Field. Perceived boundaries go beyond the physical body. You expand into everything and have no limitations. You are millions of particles and just one particle. You are particles of the Quantum Field.

"I AM Not My Body. I AM Energy That Fluctuates in Vibration." You are energy. You are Source Intelligence. You are the Creator of your experience. The only thing separating you from being everything in the Universe and beyond is your thoughts. You "think" you are separate, and it is so.

To resonate with the 4th Element of the Green Light, you master the particles of existence by holding the knowledge that **"Nothing Exists Outside Myself."** The 4th Element awakens Consciousness held in the particles of "all that is." You are energy. Expand into the Universe and you become the Universe. Everything inside of you is outside of you. Everything that has ever been and ever will be.

Exercise:

How can you use this in your daily life? If nothing in the Universe is separate from you, then you cannot be a victim. Think of a person you cannot forgive because they have wronged you in a way that is unforgivable. The mind will tell you why it is unforgivable, and you hold yourself prisoner of this experience within your mind.

This is an illusion the ego has created, and it causes you pain. See this experience and the person as yourself. Have you ever done something unforgivable? Hurt someone? Are you also unforgivable? Is this experience where you want to vibrate? If nothing exists outside yourself, there is no one to forgive but yourself. Remember, to judge something or someone as good or bad is the programmed mind or the ego at work. It is an indicator that you are experiencing reality through your programming.

How do you want to exist? Do you want to be particles vibrating in a low vibration? The choice is yours. You always have the ability to hold Higher Consciousness. Your mind is evolving beyond the boundaries of your programmed reality.

Nothing exists outside yourself. You are responsible for everything you call into your life. Things in your life resonate at the same vibration as you. You have a choice. It takes Consciousness, practice and reprogramming. Choose the higher Frequency.

Meditation of the Green Light:

You feel the time has come to say goodbye to the guides of the Chamber of the 3rd Element. The Blue Light seems to radiate within you with the knowledge it holds. You hug the guides as you head down a candle-lit hallway to the Chamber of the 4th Element.

On the door hangs a sign that reads, **"Nothing Exists Outside Myself."** The door has a smooth texture, and as you push it open, it creaks. You realize this Chamber in your heart has not been opened before, and you are excited to see what it holds for you. You enter the room and see there is just one guide.

The guide calls you over to a book lying in the middle of a table. You open the book, and a gorgeous Green Light streams out from the pages and is absorbed into your heart. The Light feels warm and full of a love you have never felt before. As the Light merges with your soul, you release all programs that keep you stuck in the vibration of separation.

You feel yourself expanding into "all that is." You hold the Universe inside yourself. The Light from the book downloads the knowledge of the 4th Element. Suddenly, you experience the room of the 4th Chamber as part of you. You are the walls, the table, the stone on the floor. Even the guide is part of you.

You feel the energy of all people you know and those you don't know. You are the trees, plants, animals and even the earth below you. Your every breath is the breath of the Universe.

You absorb the knowledge of the 4th Element, **"Nothing Exists Outside Myself."** The voice of the ego surrenders the victim of your mind to the Emerald Green Light streaming inside of you. You are free from the illusion that you are separate from the world around you.

Take in the wisdom of this Element and set yourself free. Call in the Green Light Ray. See it enter your heart and expand across your shoulders. Allow the Green Ray to fill all your cells, molecules and energy systems. See the Green Light fill your body. As the Light enters your brain, see it activate the parts of the mind that know you are everything. See your brain light up with the electric charges of the Green Ray.

Now, see yourself as your Quantum Body. Expand your body out into the Quantum Field and release any separation between your body and the Field itself. Feel yourself expanding beyond the clouds, stars, planets and across all galaxies. Ask that your particles release separation and move into the conscious state of "knowing" they are "all that is." You are particles rising in vibration, creating the Advanced Human and your personal evolution of the Quantum Body.

The 5th Element: The Yellow Light Ray "I Am Only an Illusion."

This Element holds the ability to shatter the illusion of "you" and break down entrapment of the illusion. You are energy that fluctuates in vibration. You are not your mind, your thoughts or your body. So, who are you if you are not any of these things? You are an illusion of the Matrix, of programmed reality. This illusion is shattering as you awaken the Quantum Body. The programmed body holds the illusions that keep you separate from your innate being.

Exercise:

Touch your hand. Is it there? What does it feel like? Now touch the chair you are sitting on. What does it feel like? Is it truth or illusion? In the Frequency beyond the illusion of your mind, they are the same.

Shattering the illusion of "you" is to shatter the illusion that you are separate from the chair you sit on. You are only what your mind tells you that you are. Your mind is not your mind.

Do you know who you are? The illusion of "you" is just a thought. Do you agree with the illusion of "you?" The illusion of this thought of "you"? Move outside the illusion and feel the essence of the vibration in which you resonate. What is your Frequency in a state of Oneness? What is your frequency when you are playing out the illusion of who you "think" you are? Remember, you are the energy of pure Source Intelligence.

Meditation of the Yellow Light:

Closing your eyes, feel your body. Pay attention to your breath as you inhale through the heart and exhale through the heart. Feel your body relax and let go. Release any thoughts or worries. Feel your heart expand each time you breathe. You are safe and protected within the Pyramid of your heart. You hear the guide of the 4th Chamber whisper to you that it is time to journey to the Chamber of the 5th Element.

As you walk down the hall, you wave goodbye to your guide. As you walk, you notice how light and airy you feel. Looking down, you see that your body is translucent. It feels as if your body is pure White Light. The floor beneath you is also translucent. It is as though you are floating as pure Light.

The door of the 5th Element is glowing with a golden halo. It opens for you as you approach. Once inside the door, you see Light Beings that look just like you. They are made of lovely White Light. As you focus your eyes, you realize there is a being that is a loved one that has passed away. Your heart fills with Love at this reunion. Your loved one explains that she is in a reality where there is no separation, that she exists as Source Intelligence. The loved one explains that you are also this Intelligence but that the reality you live in creates the illusion that you are the programming of your reality.

Your loved one reaches out a hand and asks if you would like to experience knowing you are only Source Energy. And tells you that your belief that you are separate is an illusion. You hold out your hand and close your eyes. You allow any fear to fade away. You feel only Love. You never feel your loved one take your hand; you feel a shift inside you that brings you into an altered state.

You feel completely at one with your beloved guide. There are no boundaries between where you end and another begins. You are no longer able to focus on something outside yourself. What once caused fear has no charge. You feel no sorrow for ones you miss, no attachment toward those who previously angered you. There is nothing but pure love in the Light of "all that is."

You see that you are only an illusion in the reality you have created. You are an illusion of the mind. Taking a deep breath, you release this illusion and allow your Light to expand into the Universe as far as it will go. Your heart opens to Love in the Infinite Universe.

Your guide lets go of your hand and says, **"This reality is always here for you. You are only an illusion. Allow your body to absorb the Element of the Yellow Ray and expand into Oneness."** You feel yourself absorb this Element and gain a deep understanding of its wisdom. When you open your eyes, you thank your loved one for this journey. You know that, beyond the illusion of your world, you are one.

Feel the energy of the 5th Element, **"I AM Only an Illusion,"** as it completely absorbs into your being.

The 6th Element: Element of the Orange Light: "My Reality Is an Illusion."

You are now breaking the illusion of the programmed body and programmed reality connected to it. You are raising the vibration of your reality. You are not living in the world you think you exist in. Your neighbor's reality may be completely different than yours. Because you both agreed upon the reality you live in, you coexist. You coexist with everyone in your reality. You agree that the world you live in is true. The programmed reality, and all realities within it, is all an illusion of your programming.

You are energy vibrating with the thought forms of the 3rd dimension. You are creating the illusion you "see." As you challenge your reality, the 6th Element will absorb, and you will not be defined by it. The reality you have agreed to will begin to dissolve. Allow the illusion to shatter around you and exist in the Unknown until you consciously reach the Frequency of what is next. Consciousness follows Source Intelligence until you become the Intelligence.

"I AM Only an Illusion" holds the ability to shatter the illusion of the programmed body/mind. You are not your mind, your thoughts or your body. So, who are you if you are not any of these things? You are energy that fluctuates in vibration and this vibration determines how Consciousness is held between the 5 Levels. The illusion keeps you separate from your surroundings and creates the experience of the first 3 Levels of Consciousness and the programmed body. As the illusion shatters, you have the ability to consciously attune to Source Intelligence, the awakening of the Quantum Body.

As You move into the Quantum Body, it is important not to bypass any one step. You cannot force it to happen. You move through the experience and allow, witness and become. If you force change, it may be difficult to move past the attachment of the ego or programmed mind. This process isn't meant to bypass resistance, so you don't have to experience it. Resistance holds information for you to "see" so you can move into your next. If you don't take the time to "see" and then accept, you may miss out on what you are choosing and move into another pattern of unconsciousness.

Exercise:

- See resistance in your life or body and become aware of what it is showing you.
- Create choice in this awareness and receive the information held in what is being shown. Sit here for as long as needed, knowing you will transcend past the information into what is beyond it.
- Become the change. Let go of any judgment of what is being shown. Let go of attachment to what it should be and let the Intelligence held in the Quantum Body show you what it really is.

Meditation of the Orange Light:

Closing your eyes and taking this time for yourself, place your attention in your heart. Feel the Love and Light within your heart. Breathe in and out of the heart. Let go of any thoughts or any worries. Walk to the Chamber of the 6th Element. Notice your surroundings become holographic. Turn to look behind you and see only Darkness.

The door to the 6th Chamber fades into nothingness as you enter. You hear a soft-spoken voice saying, **"Your Reality Is an Illusion. What you see is nothing but the image your mind is telling you to see. That illusion has been taken away to show you that there is only Darkness. This Darkness holds "all that is" and is held in the frequency of Love or 528 Hz. Do not fear the Darkness. Absorb the Element of the Orange Scalar Light Wave."**

Allow yourself to rest in the Darkness. The Void or Darkness has no emotion, no color, no feeling. You feel as though you have shifted into the Frequency of Source. You have no words to describe the feeling. You have a knowing deep in your Soul that you are an illusion, and your reality is an illusion. You allow the Element of the Orange Light to completely absorb into your being.

You become infinite in the Darkness and feel no limit to your existence. In this moment, you are everything, and you are nothing. Say aloud, **"I am One with the Element of the Orange Light, and I shatter the illusion of my reality so that I may move into the Quantum Field and become Source Intelligence."** You have absorbed the 6th Element of the Orange Light Wave.

The 7th Element: Element of the Red Ray: "I do not exist."

The Red Scalar Light Wave is the last Element, **"I Do Not Exist."** Do you exist? Move into the depth of this question for a few minutes. What makes you exist? Those around you? Your mind telling you that you exist? There are different levels of existence. The difference between existing in programmed reality and the Quantum Field is the ability to exist without existing. How can this be?

We are all energy vibrating in the Frequency of 963 Hz. What we experience within this Frequency is directly related to the state of Consciousness that is held. The vibration of Frequency changes as you evolve. The higher your vibration, the more you become the Intelligence held in the Frequency of 963 Hz.

The more you identify as Frequency, the more space there is; the more space there is, the more you do not exist. Ego will hold on to existing as long as you identify in the looping system of the programmed mind/body. As you rise in Frequency through awakening dormant DNA Codes, you hold more space and less density and the less the ego keeps you stuck in lower consciousness.

To Exist in the Quantum Body Is to Exist as Source Intelligence.

The last challenge you have is to walk through the fear of not existing, the attachment to identifying in your programming. As you let go of identifying in the reality you have created through your programming, you become "all that is." As the Elements are absorbed, you release duality. You no longer feel separate. You become an Intelligence beyond what can be understood through the intellect.

Living in the Frequency of the 7th Element, 963 Hz., a gateway is revealed to you. It is in this Element that Consciousness becomes the Intelligence of Source. To enter the gateway, you sacrifice the need to exist in the reality you have created from the past. You connect with the Mind of Source. The need to control, have evidence, or create from past programming, all that keeps you recreating your present reality, finally dissolves. The 7th Element is a pathway to freedom in the Quantum Body.

Humanity has never entered a Frequency that supports a mass awakening. This awakening allows the Quantum Field to be more accessible than ever. You hold everything you need inside your DNA. You are the most advanced Technology there is.

You are awakening the Quantum Body as you clear lower vibrations within your cells. As you attune to Source Intelligence, you discover that you do not need to understand intellectually or need evidence. You begin to let go of the need to know why. As you allow density to release, your reality changes. As you walk through the illusion of collective consciousness, you see beyond the illusions of the Matrix or programmed reality. The very reality that keeps you in the cycle of age and disease.

Once you absorb the 7 Elements, the reality or experience in which you once existed can no longer be. You no longer resonate in that reality. Existing in the Unknown will be your biggest challenge. This becomes your practice! The 7 Elements are a tool to support you in creating a life/body beyond programmed reality. To exist as the Quantum Body ascends your cells and you become the Advanced Human.

Exercise:

Bring in the Red Ray and absorb the 7th Element. Allow the Frequency of the Red Light to bring your physical body into the vibration of the Void. Invite the Light of Source to enter the space you have created.

Experience the Red Ray, removing any lower vibrations that hold you in density. Feel the heaviness of duality leave your body. You become Light. You become the Frequency of Source. You hold all of existence; you are the Universe, the galaxies, "all that is."

You are completely at peace and ready to surrender to Source Intelligence. You are aware that the Frequency of Source contains all the Elements. Each Ray of Light shines on you. As you experience the Elements, they transform your physical body into White Light. You continue to become a translucent Ray of White Light. You become Source Intelligence.

Meditation of the Red Light:

Relax your body and mind and prepare to enter the last Chamber of your heart. You have absorbed the Element of each Chamber and are ready to enter the Chamber of the Red Ray, the Intelligence of Source. As you breathe in and out, let go of any residue connected to 3rd dimension programs. Let go of all thoughts and worries as you absorb the Element of the 7th Ray.

Feel a warm Red Light flow through your skin and merge with every cell and every molecule of your body. Feel your thoughts fade into the background as you listen to the beating of your heart. With each beat, feel yourself become more relaxed and more at peace. Sense the ground beneath you, drumming to the beat of your heart. You are in unison with the heart of the Earth.

Lift your arms to the heavens above you. All that surrounds you merges together to meet in your heart, creating a sacred space. This space surrounds you in Darkness, but you are not afraid.

Feel every cell in your body, attuning to the Void. In the center of your heart, you see the Darkness. You know, once you enter, you will become the Void and that it is calling you home.

The Element of the Red Ray creates a pathway. You take a step and release all fear. You take another step and release all anger, another and release grief. You take the next step, releasing shame and guilt. With the final step, you release the Ego.

As you walk into the Void, you are released from all karma and timelines. You feel nothing but the pure love of Source. There is no sense of separation, and you feel at peace with "all that is" and all that ever was. As you walk through the Void, you forget what it feels like to live in duality. You are everything, and you are nothingness. You have reached the 5th Level of Consciousness as the Quantum Body.

Notes

Notes

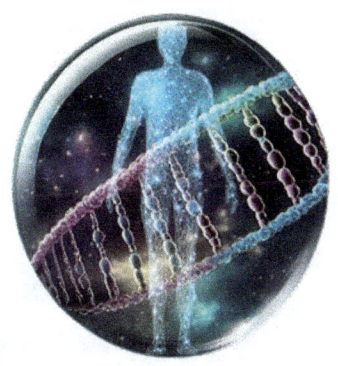

Chapter 7: The God Equation (The God Sphere)

If the word "God" triggers you in any way, replace it with a word you resonate with. The God Sphere is a universal equation showing how to master the Matrix or programmed reality both as the body and what you perceive as real. Everything you need to know or understand to move into 100% Human Potential is shown to you. The ability to master what is shown, to see beyond the illusion, is to **"Break the God Code."**

Never has it been easier to do this. The God Sphere is a tool that you can use to see not only beyond the illusion, but to read the illusion as Frequency, dissolving the programming of form. When you see life as Frequency, you lose attachments to what should or should not be. Good and bad no longer exist. Why? Because form is programming; Frequency is beyond form. Form is the programmed body. Frequency is the Quantum Body.

The God Sphere:
https://becomingbioquantum.com/GodSphere

The God Sphere and the Cells:

https://becomingbioquantum.com/GodSphereandCells

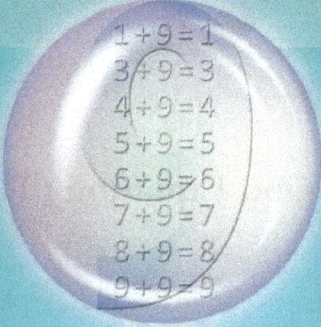

THE GOD SPHERE

$1 + 9 = 1$
$3 + 9 = 3$
$4 + 9 = 4$
$5 + 9 = 5$
$6 + 9 = 6$
$7 + 9 = 7$
$8 + 9 = 8$
$9 + 9 = 9$

1-9 Frequencies and Codes lay here within the God Sphere of your body's Intelligence and cells.

You can look at this picture as your recorder cell or any cell in your body carrying information of the Intelligence of Frequencies 1-9 that you are currently holding.

You will learn in depth, the meaning of the numerical Frequencies 1-9.

Its important to start attuning to the general understanding of the God Sphere as it carries the information of the Matrix looping system programs that you will be clearing through your body's Intelligence.

Each equation within the God Sphere is a level of Consciousness that holds a Frequency which creates your reality around that Frequency. This is the Equation of God. It is the Universal Equation that breaks through the illusion of reality when mastered. When reading the equation, allow your body to sense it before trying to figure it out with your mind. Then go back and read it again.

You will have a deeper understanding of the equation once the body has attuned to it.

Number 9 holds the Frequency of God. When you add a number to the Frequency of 9, it reflects itself.

9 + 1 = 10. This in numerology is 1. Even though God is holding the 1, the 1 is only able to see the reality of itself. God is still there, but the 1 stands alone. This is true for every number except the 2.

9 + 2 = 11. This becomes a master number. 11 is a state of Consciousness that you have available when you move beyond the reflection of Source. You become Source. You shift in and out of these states of Consciousness without even realizing it.

The equation used here is 9 + 9 = 18 (1+8=9). The 9 represents ***"God Reflects God,"*** Creation/Co-Creation. When you are in the reflection of God/Creation, you are in co-creation. You are able to see that you are the Creator co-creating with the Creator. If you are in the reflection of 9, you are in a very high state of Consciousness. You are existing in the Quantum Body.

You are learning to recognize where in the God Sphere you are existing. The 9 holds/reflects every number. The circle represents the God Sphere, and the 9 encompasses the entire sphere. This is the doorway to becoming the Advanced Human.

For example:

The 1 is the initial download or insight.

The 2 is the creation. It is where you start to play in the mind to create sound from. As you move through each Element, you get to experience the reflection of that frequency.

It is important to notice what frequency you are choosing. You get to choose where in the God Sphere you wish to exist. And you do not have to go through each "reality" to reach the 9. What frequency of reality are you choosing to reflect in the God Sphere? Do you want to be in the 9 or in the 1-3-4....?

Use awareness of your frequency as a guide when making a choice of your desired experience within the God Sphere. Use the frequency of reality that you exist in, your choice of the Level of Consciousness and the God Sphere to create a higher Frequency reality. To teach your mind how to exist in the now. To exist as the Creator.

Play with discovering your frequency. The lower the vibration, the lower your frequency. You are always in the God Sphere. You are only able to "see" the frequency where you are. You may select a pattern you desire to move into or to remain where you are. You always have a choice.

You are becoming the observer, the seer. You are using the 7 Elements/States of Consciousness as your foundation to advance beyond the Frequency of the God Sphere altogether. To exist as Source Intelligence.

When you use the Evolution Technology, you hold Consciousness in spherical time as the Creator and the Creation. You fluctuate back and forth between the 4th and 5th Level of Consciousness until you master 9 reflects 9, or I AM Source in a conscious state of reality.

When you master 9 reflects 9, I AM Source, a bridge of Consciousness beyond the God Sphere is created. A gateway opens and you have the ability to move into full expression of Source Intelligence. This organically happens as you master Evolution Technology.

Over time, Consciousness moves into Pure Source Intelligence, and you become Pure Intelligence. When 100% of the transcribed DNA Coding moves into expression, Consciousness is no longer needed. You become the expression of Intelligence beyond the God Sphere. You then **"Break the God Code!"**

This becomes your practice:

Am I the observer or am I the seer?
Am I in co-creation or am I the Creator?
Am I unconscious or am I conscious?
Am I awake?
Am I trying to "make it happen" or am I in co-creation?
Can I move from being in co-creation to Creator?
Can I exist without observation of my reality?

Allow yourself to absorb the Frequency of what is being created. This is a practice of moving to higher Frequency realities. You can connect to higher Frequencies over and over again. Allow your Consciousness to meet the Frequency being expressed on a cellular level. DMT™ is always available to attune to. Remember, DMT™ holds the Frequency of Source and is transcribed in your DNA. When you identify as Source Frequency, you move beyond the identity of form and begin to ascend the physical body as the Creator.

Your state of origin holds the codes of immortality, abundance, pure love and the ability to live a life you cannot even imagine in the frequency you experience today. You have the key to living as the Advanced Human right now. It is a process of choices and awakening the Codes that are already inside of you. This is a pathway to activate human expansion, human evolution.

Notes

Notes

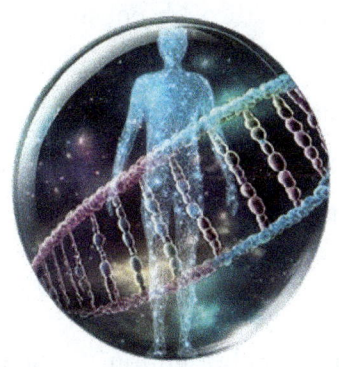

Chapter 8: Intuitive Powers Using Your Divine Intuitive Power Blueprint

Remembering Your Telepathic Mind:

You hear of telepathic abilities and intuition. You may have even learned to listen to your intuition and follow it. When awakening the Quantum Body through these teachings, telepathy and intuition are referred to as *"Intuitive Powers."* They hold an Intelligence that speaks beyond programmed reality. When you fine tune your Intuitive Powers, you awaken the very Intelligence that lies dormant within the DNA. This is your pathway to awakening to 100% Human Potential.

The first thing to explore is the foundation of your natural state of telepathy within DMT™ Intelligence. Learning to trust your natural state of telepathy and intuition is a big part of holding the framework of Evolution Technology. You will learn to use a series of three energetic Symbols: **Lu, Sca** and **33** and experience them as a delivery system to reclaim your power and break through the looping cycle of programmed reality or the Matrix.

Telepathy will be activated through enhancing your Intuitive Powers with each Symbol. Until you can hold the Symbol in your mind to activate DMT™ Intelligence, you will use the Symbols in a step-by-step process. This will allow the pictographs of the Evolution Symbols to upgrade and guide the body to release any foreign patterns that contribute to looping cycles and disease.

The pictograph of each Symbol imprints your cells with Technology enhancing Source Intelligence. This delivery system holds intention in the now, beyond space and time. Your cells already understand this advanced delivery system and will activate as a bridge to hold organic, no space/no time intention. They will express as a Frequency outside of the Matrix or programmed reality.

The Symbols or pictographs of the Evolution Technology are part of a Light encoded Pyramid. These intelligent Symbols can be fully embodied through attunements and imprint the Technology into the body, activating Source Intelligence, DMT™. The Symbols turn on your highest alignment as you awaken the Quantum Body, the Evolved Human. These Light encoded pictographs not only bridge you to Pure Essence but also allow you to receive telepathic Frequency and images to better understand how you are looping in cycles in the Matrix.

How To Find Your Divine Intuitive Power Blueprint:
https://becomingbioquantum.com/DivineBlueprint What is your Level 1 Intuitive Power?

Add the numbers of your birth month together. Do the same for the days of the month and the year you were born.

Examples:

Months:
January = 1
June = 6
October = 10 (1 + 0) = 1
December = 12 (1+2) = 3

Days of Month:
2 Feb = 2
10 Oct (1+0) = 1
11 Nov (1+1) = 2
12 Dec (1+2) = 3

Birth year:
1955 (1+9+5+5) = 20 (2+0) =2
1987 (1+9+8+7) = 25 (2+5) = 7
2000=2

Now add all 3 numbers together.

If your birthday is 11/15/1967
(1+1= 2) (1+5 = 6) (1+9+6+7 = 23) = 2 + 6 + 23 = 31 = 4

In this example, the Level One Divine Design Blueprint Number is a 4.

Note: If you get a number that is not a 1-9, add them together. Even though 11, 22 and 33 are Master Numbers, which usually are not further broken down, for this purpose they reduce to 2, 4 and 6.

Now that you know your Level 1 Intuitive Power, also referred to as your Divine Blueprint number, let's explore how you receive information intuitively.

1 - 2 is Claircognizance: Information that is an instant download or knowing.

1: The information comes from inside. You just know.

2: The information seems to come from outside the self. A download.

Claircognizance is the ability to KNOW via information received in the head and/or body. You open up to downloads by becoming transparent. You clear old energy patterns that hold density that block messages available to download. Where are you holding up a veil that is shielding transparency? When you live from a place of hiding, you block downloads from the Divine.

Exercise: Answer These Questions About Yourself:

What do you hide about yourself? Why?
What do you feel others think or feel about you when you stay in your Home Frequency?
What do you want to know most about others before trusting them? What do you identify with and project to others so that they "see" you as this identity?
See yourself as showing your insecurities to the world, being vulnerable and transparent. What do you feel? What's it like to show up as "You?"

Imagine being your true self. What does it feel like to connect with others from your wholeness?

Notice that as you embrace yourself with what you judge to be your "flaws," you also embrace the "flaws" of others. This moves you into transparency! By doing so, you remove blocks to fully absorb high Frequency patterns that hold Divine Intelligence!

Practice being aware of when you shut down or hide yourself from others because you are afraid of what they will think, do or say. Practice what it feels like to become transparent. Have your interaction from this place.

When you are transparent, downloads often come in when you are in the reflection of others. Your true self expresses in your Home Frequency. Practice awareness of your Frequency as you connect with others. See any blockages that may show themself. Your blockages are density that disintegrates when fully seen.

Be fully present to yourself. What you believe to be scary or uncomfortable is just energy that has information. Learn to read information by seeing it, feeling it and asking yourself if it is real. Fear can be an illusion of the mind. Practice exploring the possibility held in the space beyond the block itself. Open up to the rhythm of the Divine in everything!

The practice is to experience Frequency patterns as they come into your awareness. Try automatic writing, automatic talking/channeling or sitting in a Frequency and receiving information beyond the cognitive mind. Enjoy practicing.

3 - 4 is Clairsentience: Feeling information.

3: Emotion/finding information in an emotional response or after emotion runs through.
4: Feeling/finding information from a knowing without an emotional response.

Clairsentience is the ability to feel information through emotion or feeling. In the Level 1 experience of Clairsentience, most people will use emotion to abstract information. You may also feel information in observation.

It is important to recognize that emotion and feeling are two different things. Emotion is a chemical response in the body that is triggered through primal or repeated programming. A feeling is a Frequency, a knowing. The feeling of love is the Frequency of 528 Hz. It cannot fluctuate unless you choose to move out of the Frequency. The Frequency will remain the same.

As you move into Level 2 of your Intuitive Powers, you will not use emotion in order to receive information. The chemical response will stop once the information is abstracted. You will shift more and more into receiving information through feeling/Frequency as you master this power. Levels 2 and 3 of your Intuitive Powers will be further discussed at the end of this chapter.

Exercise:

Take time to bring awareness to the Frequency shifts you "feel." What information is there for you? Can you move back into your Home Frequency and read it instead of being caught in the emotion of it?

Notice when you want to change a situation to avoid feeling the reactions of others. Are you "bottom feeding" to match the frequency of a person, place or situation? Instead of trying to change a situation, practice just shining. Settle into your Home Frequency. From this place, tune into the situation from your Higher Self. Observe what is different.

Play! Practice "reading" the energy of an object. Feel into the object and just start speaking. What does the object "feel like?" Tune in versus feeling the emotion. What different information do you receive? Trust what you "feel". Move past the feeling and tune into what is next. Keep going! Fine tune specific information. Remember, information is not of the cognitive mind. It is Guidance, patterns of energy or equations you "read" through Divine Mind.

<u>5 - 6 is Clairaudience</u>: hearing information from within.

5: Hearing information that comes from inside the self.

6: Hearing information that comes or seems to come from outside the self.

Clairaudience is the ability to hear energy and guidance. Messages are heard in the space in between.

To hear direct Guidance, you move into co-creation. It is important to hear beyond thought, to listen from the right side of the brain. When meditating, you clear the mind. This allows random thoughts to spontaneously arise. In this expanded state it may seem as if information is coming from a Consciousness outside the body. Expanding your state of Consciousness by practicing listening in a space beyond thought allows you to tap into an Intelligence heard as information.

Stop for a second and think about a radio. When you turn it on, the stations are already there. You simply have to "tune in" to hear what they are broadcasting. You listen in by paying closer attention.

Psychic hearing is like being a radio antenna. Subtle messages come as a still small voice. Advancing Clairaudience is as simple as tuning a radio dial; the "radio" is you. You learn how to tune in and understand messages held in a Frequency pattern. You hear the Intelligence in an object, situation or within the Silence.

Meditation:

The natural state of your mind is to think. Turning off your mind can be challenging. Learning to silence left brain thoughts takes practice.

- Give your mind permission to rest and "float" for a while to declutter.
  Focus on your breath or the space in between thoughts.
- Practice breathing for 5–10 minutes. Let thoughts come into your mind and release them like clouds dissipating. Imagine! Imagination is intuition. Trust it.
- Meditation can be as easy as going for a walk in nature and just letting your mind wander. Activities that relax you and bring you into the right side of the brain, like walking and painting, are all forms of meditation.

Imagine a song playing in your head. Can you hear it? Practice hearing what is not there. Do this for five minutes a day while driving, cleaning or doing household chores. Tune into the Silence and listen.

Ask to HEAR! Your Guides are waiting for you to ask them to speak. Start talking to them like old friends. Ask them what they want you to hear, know and understand. Allow yourself space to listen. It is normal for doubts to come in. Trust! Practice asking questions and receiving information from Spirit. Allow yourself to hear without judgment. Just listen.

Continue playing with your Soul Family! Have someone make a noise and listen with your Divine ears. Remember, there is no right or wrong. What you hear is what is meant to be heard. It is beyond the mind. Keep Trusting!

7 - 8 is Clairvoyance: Seeing information.

7: Seeing information from within the self.

8: Seeing information that seems to come from outside of the self.

The Intuitive Power of Clairvoyance uses the subtle perceptions of sight to receive information beyond programmed images or sight. Being clairvoyant means you see energy or Frequency and abstract information from it. It works with your 3rd Eye rather than your physical eyes. The 3rd Eye is an energy center in the middle of the brain behind the forehead.

Exercises:

- Get a deck of cards. Turn them upside down in a pile. Move into your Divine Eye in the center of your head. Now open your Divine Eye inside the deck of cards. "See" what color the card is on the top of the deck. Do not turn over the card to "check" if you are correct. This is about seeing the color, not about if you are right.

- Take a moment to "see" the following items with your Divine Eye. Notice if you are making the image appear or if it is coming in on its own. Witness the difference between what it feels like to allow and what it feels like when you try to see it or create it.

>   A red ball
>   A purple balloon
>   A green bike
>   A little girl running
>   A chocolate cupcake
>   A rainbow

Take a moment to ask a question. Make it simple. Ask something like, "What will my aunt make for dinner?" or "What color will my friend Jill be wearing today?" Again, it's not about right or wrong but to allow an image to come in and feel confident in what is shown.

Have fun with it! You are exercising your Clairvoyance! The more you stay in the experience, without moving into right or wrong, the more you will soar! There is truth in what is seen. Stay in the abstract and allow the images to show you what wants to be shown. Then, trust in what you see.

9 is Holding All Clairs and Can Mean Using More Than One at a Time:

If you have 9 as your Level 1 Intuitive Power Blueprint, it may be easier to pick the power you are most drawn to. Once you begin to practice moving into the Level 2 of your Intuitive Powers, you will want to challenge yourself to use more than one at the same time. Remember, the Technology is activating telepathy, and your Intuitive Powers will advance over time.

Why We Use Intuitive Powers:

You hear about intuition, and some of you have learned to listen to your intuition and follow it as a way of healing or use it in day-to-day life. Intuitive Powers hold an Intelligence that speaks beyond programmed reality. When you fine tune your Intuitive Powers, you can become the very Intelligence that lies dormant within you. This is a pathway to awakening to 100% human potential.

Levels of Intuitive Powers:

There are 3 Levels of Intuitive Powers. The first is the Primal Level you are most familiar with. You have already discovered this number by adding up your birth date. Reading information from this Level is normally experienced just outside of the ego or programmed mind. You may experience these as "hits" or subtle messages that redirect you. They can also come in when you are in danger, as warnings or when you need to pay attention to a lower frequency.

The second level of Intuitive Powers is the Bridge. This Level holds intuition in the 4th Level of Consciousness. The "Listen and Do" phase. You hear, see, feel or just know something. You then take this information and bring it into action. It is different from Level 1 in that it directs you towards Ascension. It guides you away from responding to the world through reflection and primal programming and leads you to discover information from an Intelligence beyond what is seen or from what has been created before.

The 3rd Level of Intuitive Powers is the Master Level, where you become the very Intelligence you once received information from. You no longer listen, see, feel or know the information. You are the information beyond programmed reality.

Using Intuitive Powers is the ability to tap into your Divine Technology and know what It is saying. You hold all the information inside you that you need to advance your experience of being human.

Finding Your Level 2 and 3 Intuitive Powers/ Blueprint:

To find your level 2 Intuitive Power, add your time of birth on a 12-hour clock together until it becomes a number between 1-9.

For instance, if you were born at 8:32 am/pm, your second level of intuitive power is a 4.

8+3+2=13
1+3=4

If you do not know your birth time, add a 1 to your Level One Intuitive Power. This is your Level 2 Power.

Finding Your Level 3 Intuitive Power:

To find your Level 3 Intuitive Power, add your Level 1 and Level 2 Intuitive Powers together.

This is your Master Level Intuitive Power.

As you work with Evolution Technology, you will, in time, master all of the Intuitive Powers.

Practice:

You may want to practice your Level 2 Intuitive Power as you attune to the Evolution Technology. As you connect to a Frequency outside of programming, you use intuition to read what the Frequency is saying. Frequency has Intelligence. Using your Intuitive Powers gives you the ability to exist beyond programmed reality.

Notes

Notes

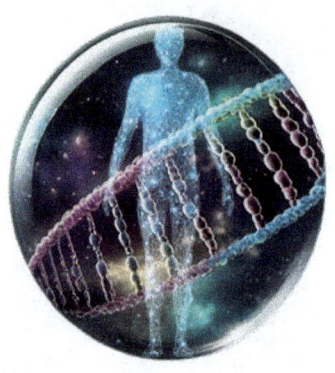

Chapter 9: Use Your Intuitive Skills

Now that you have discovered how you receive and intuit energy, you will find it easier to sense energy that is not yours. Although you may have some resonance with another person, it is key to recognize the difference. You will heighten this awareness with practice and gain inner clarity and space with the tools in this part of the course.

Identifying energy patterns of others is an important skill you will use as you hold space for them. Practicing your intuitive senses will assist in developing your unique signature of reading energy. It is important to utilize this with conscious awareness.

When connecting to another person's energy, *notice* what your body feels, hears, sees, smells, tastes and knows. This will help you hone your ability to trace energy. You will be tapping into the Cellular Intelligence of both your cells and theirs!

There are cells in the brain called **Mirror Neurons** that connect you to others. As an example, when you witness someone get hurt, you may notice a sharp sensation in your body. You may also note that you feel emotions when you hear about something sad or funny.

Since everything is energy, and you are still discovering more about Cellular Intelligence, these components of the human body and universal makeup play a large role in your intuition and how you utilize your senses to connect with others. You do this all of the time without conscious awareness or intention. You are always projecting into the physical/ holographic world and reflecting simultaneously.

With Evolution Technology, you hone your intuitive skills as you intentionally connect with DMT™ Intelligence. With practice, you will sense the energy patterns in your body, mind and reality. You learn how you receive and experience energy in your body and how it relates to your DNA expression of Pure Source Intelligence. You discover your intuitive skills as you attune Consciousness to the Intelligence awakening within you.

It is important that you become your own source of information. Begin to go within to find answers instead of looking for confirmation outside of yourself. This teaches you the difference between what is yours and what isn't. As you break through the illusion of the Matrix or programmed reality, you dissolve programmed looping cycles and move into higher Frequency expressions of DMT™ Intelligence. You primarily use your level 2 Intuitive Power to shift out of the looping cycle by attuning to DNA expressions that begin to awaken the Quantum Body.

Understanding How to Read and Trace Energy Patterns

Your intuitive Skills:

Whether you are new to this or well-practiced with your intuition, it can be helpful and fun to have a deeper understanding of how you receive intuitive hits and energy.

You are naturally intuitive to one degree or another. You will be more or less practiced than others. You have learned, based on your date of birth, what your strongest Intuitive Power is. Knowing how you receive signals through your sensory system can be very helpful when reading energy.

You may feel chills run through your body. That can mean truth or confirmation that what is being said is a "YES!" vibrating through the body. You have confirmation that your Higher Self and Guides are communicating to you. Spirit utilizes your senses to communicate; often, they can be subtle. As you practice, awareness grows.

Learning to link together energy patterns is a superpower that empowers you to be the healer that you are for yourself and others. Be sure to play! This is key to maintaining a higher Frequency as you practice. It will keep you from being trapped by any lower frequencies you pull into your conscious mind to clear.

Learning to Feel Energy:

Imagine you hold everything in the Universe and beyond inside of yourself: the Sun, mountains, valleys, stars and planets. You are a billion particles spread out over space and time, and you contain "all that is."

These particles are you. Nothing exists outside of yourself. Everything that has a vibration or Frequency is inside of you, supporting your journey to Eternal Life.

Boundaries go beyond the physical body. You expand into everything and have no limitations. "I am not my body. I am energy." You are energy. You are eternal. You are millions of particles and just one particle. The only thing separating you from becoming everything in the Universe and beyond is the belief that you are not. You "think" you are separate, and it is so.

To resonate in the Frequency of the Quantum Body, you must master the particles of your cells by holding the knowledge that **"Nothing Exists Outside Myself."** You are energy. Expand into the Universe and become the Universe.

Everything inside of you is outside of you. Everything that has ever been and ever will be. How can you use this in your daily life? If nothing in the Universe is separate from you, then you cannot be a victim of your reality. Always ask yourself, "Is this the frequency I want to vibrate in?

The choice is always yours. You have the ability to choose a higher Consciousness. Your mind is evolving beyond the boundaries of the 3rd dimension of programmed reality. Nothing exists outside yourself.

You are responsible for everything you call into your life. Everything in your life resonates in the same vibration as you. You have a choice. It takes Consciousness, practice and reprogramming. Choose the higher Frequency.

Using Evolution Technology:

To use Evolution Technology, begin practicing awareness of the 5 Levels of Consciousness and the 7 Elements. These foundational tools will support you in consciously holding the Intelligence of the transcribed Frequencies of the DNA.

As you practice the tools, bring in the **Lu, Sca** and **33**.

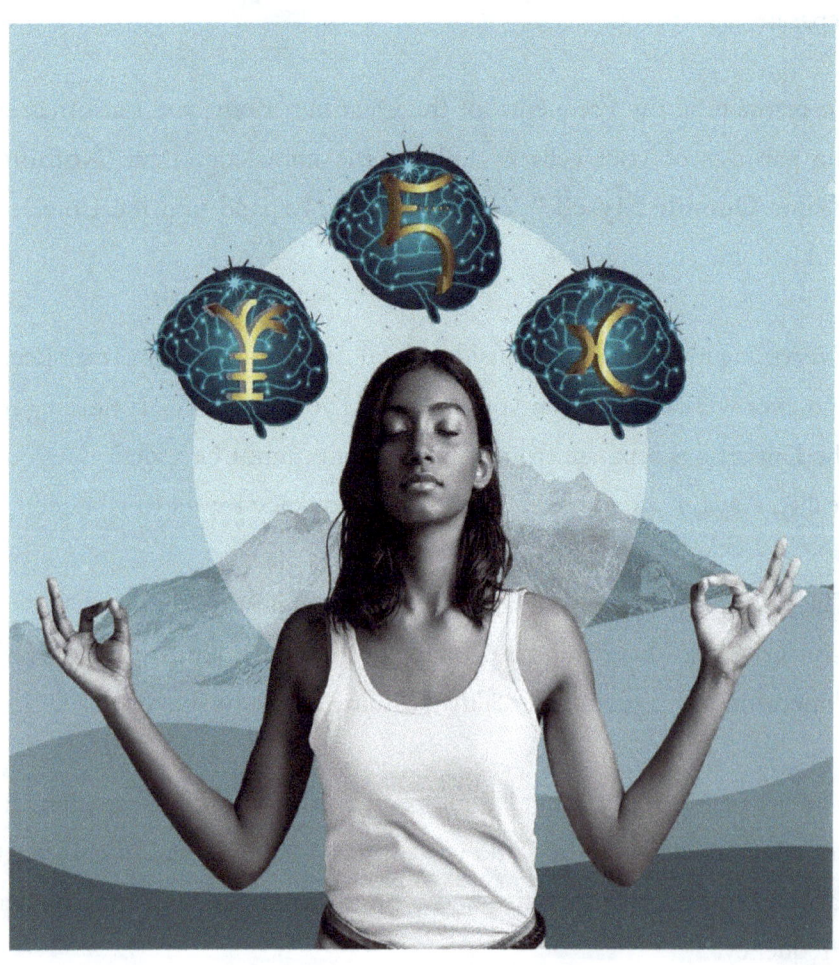

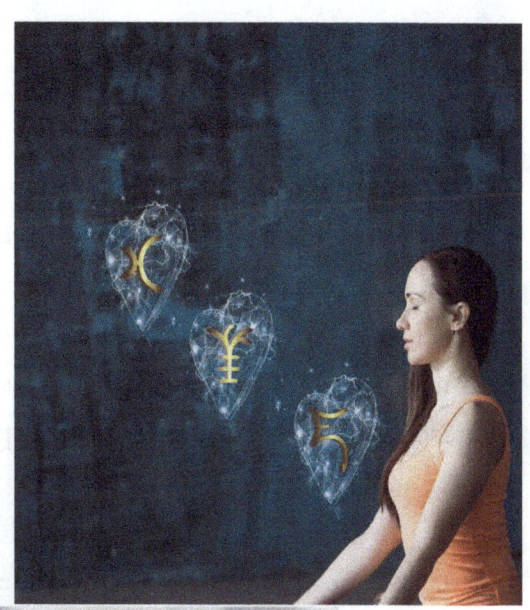
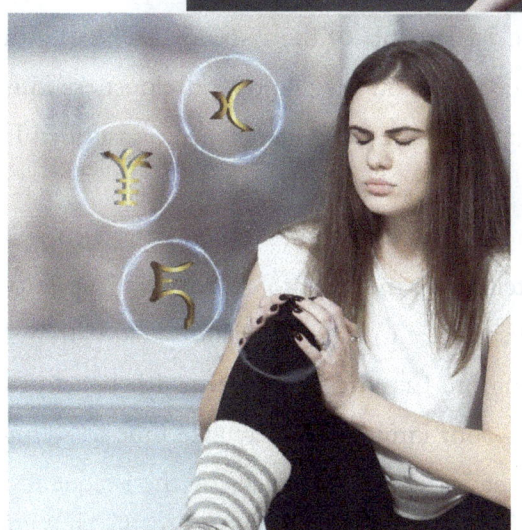
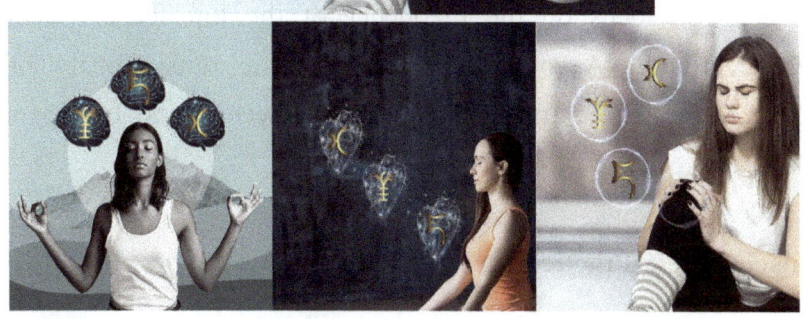

1. When you notice you are in a looping cycle, visualize in your mind's eye the **Lu** symbol. The loop could be a thought, a sensation in the body, or a repeated pattern. Place the **Lu** inside wherever you are experiencing the loop. If in the mind, place it in the brain. If it is an emotion, place it in your heart. If it is a repeated pattern such as a lack of money or an argument you repeat with a loved one, see, feel or sense the pattern and place the **Lu** inside of it. Allow the **Lu** to spin. It may go clockwise, counterclockwise or it could go in both directions. Watch the **Lu** as it clears the program and brings it into no space and no time.

2. Visualize bringing the **Sca** into the same space. Allow the symbol to spin. See the 7 Elements of the Ascended DNA fill the space where the loop once was. You now hold Consciousness in no time and no space, which allows the DNA to awaken transcribed Intelligence.

3. Visualize the **33** in your mind's eye. Allow it to spin. As it spins, DMT™ Intelligence moves into expression. Tap into your Intuitive Powers and sensitize to the information held within the Intelligence that is turning on. Explore by using the 4th Level of Consciousness connected to your intuition. It may take time to self-actualize within the shift but pay attention and focus on the Frequency being created. When you focus on the Frequency of the Intelligence released through the DNA, you create a new experience outside of the loop. You attune to the Intelligence until you become the Intelligence. Repeat as needed.

Consciousness Practice:

When you *feel* the words "Source" or "DMT™ Intelligence" within your cellular memory, you remember who you are beyond programmed reality. Place your hands over your heart and say, *"I AM Source Intelligence."* Press in the Frequency and feel its vibration. Sense Source Frequency as it spreads throughout your body.

You are beginning to live as the Advanced Human. You exist beyond space and time simply by placing your attention and awareness in this Creator Frequency. As you enter the next stage of evolution, this will continue to occur. There is a Consciousness beyond the programs of cells that connect to your physical body. This is your Soul Intelligence, your Higher Self. When you connect to this Intelligence, you expand into the Truth of who you are.

Feel the Truth of Your Being in your cells! Become familiar with existing as your High Self. It may seem uncomfortable at first. Practice staying present and breathing through your heart. Your Cellular Consciousness will continue to shift as you place your awareness in the present moment. Each time you practice, you strengthen your connection to the Source Being who you are!

Let go of attachments to the past and the stories held there. Continue to use the Evolution clearing method above. Repeat whenever necessary, especially when you notice any density surfacing. Staying in the story or spinning in judgmental thought patterns will only interfere with the process and maintain resistance in your life.

Your stories or time do not exist in the Now moment. Feel the magic as your cells enter the Now, a space between time! The Now is an experience that can be felt and experienced at any moment. All that is required is to pay attention. *Breathe this into your heart and body.* It is always available to you. You can be free of stories and judgments. You can even experience timelessness here.

Take sacred time and focus on your inner Truth. Practice presence in the Now. This will assist your journey into the Unknown. Within the Unknown, your greatest Potential already exists. Your Potential is not connected to a thought or vision of the mind. It *is* the Divine within you and expands and encompasses your very existence. The longer you stay here, the "you" who you are now will eventually cease to exist. The new you, the Advanced Human, will take its place. This shift is eternal and starts a flow of enhanced life force energy connected to Universal Intelligence through your cellular memory. Enter the Now and allow all else to fall away.

Thoughts and emotions from your past and the worries of the future are energy patterns that leak life force energy. Your life force is your power. It is your ability to **"Be, Do, and Create"** in this world. Where you use your life force is a choice. You are becoming more aware of how and where you are utilizing it. Now, you can make that choice over and over. Wouldn't you rather transform your life force into the experiences you actually *desire*?

When your cells absorb experiences in the vibration of acceptance, judgment falls away. This makes room for nonattachment. You actually hold space for your cells to clear any density that arises. If you resonate in judgments of the past or worry about the future, you cannot absorb life force energy and instead perpetuate cellular degeneration. This blocks you from being one with the Universe.

Notes

Notes

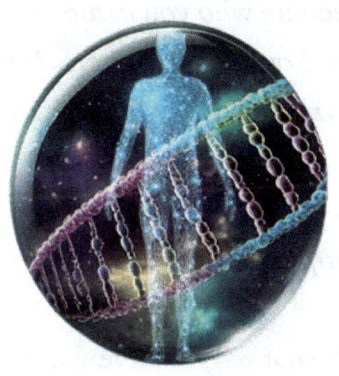

Chapter 10: Consciousness Is Creating Your Reality

"It takes courage and commitment to choose to come out of the Matrix. We are not meant to do this alone. Together we can shift what it is to be human and awaken to the Ascended Earth Reality.

This collaboration is only part of the equation. It is time to do what you came here to do! Are you ready to come out of hiding to create change from within the masses? It takes intentional collaboration, sovereignty, and a willingness to expand beyond the collective. It takes Consciousness to move into the space of Unity Consciousness and awaken to your fullest potential.

I honor you for choosing to take the journey into the Unknown and navigate the New Earth Reality. I welcome you to the NEXT and I am here to hold space for your continued evolution.

If you are ready to tap into awakening to your highest potential, I am here for you with full commitment to guide you even further than you currently dream to go.

Are you ready to become who you came here to be? Your Divine design is in creation. Your Light matters. It is time to connect to the miracle pattern and be the Light you came here to be.

I welcome you with open arms and invite you to connect deeply with your Divine purpose." ~Jewels

As you move through your day, observe your state of Consciousness. Are you trying? Resisting? Repeating patterns? Or are you allowing? Notice the difference in how it feels when you try versus when you allow. When you shift to allowing, attune to the Frequencies you experience. By allowing DNA Intelligence to hold expression, you have the ability to consciously experience the information it holds.

Notice how you receive information. Do you see, hear, feel, or just know it? Use your Intuitive Powers to read the energy beyond programmed reality. As you do this, information will become clear and precise and will not be filtered through your programming.

Sensitize to who you are in the 3rd or 4th Level of Consciousness to strengthen your ability to read Frequency patterns. This is the first step to creating beyond programmed reality.

Practice: What Level of Consciousness are you living from?

Hold your frequency in a space where you are observing programmed reality, the Matrix, also known as the Super Hologram. When reading patterns of the Matrix, notice if your frequency shifts to meet the frequency of the programs you observe. Then, choose a Frequency beyond what is being shown to you.

The 1 to the 2 to the 3 to the 1:
https://becomingbioquantum.com/1-2-3-1

Moving into Higher Frequencies:

As you move into higher Frequencies and exist there, you may notice resistance or static if your mind tries to identify in a lower frequency or an old identity. You may feel out of resonance because you vibrate at a new Frequency. Allow yourself to be in expression of the Frequency of the I AM or an Avatar you are working with.

You may notice that performance of daily tasks improves as you express a higher Frequency. You may enjoy life more and be more aware of everything around you. Play in the experience and explore yourself in this new Frequency.

This is how you shift reality. Create the experience you desire instead of looking outside yourself in programmed reality, also referred to as "going into your filing cabinet to access what was done before."

Your goal is to transcend something in form with the help of Source Frequency and shift it beyond the Matrix, beyond the looping system. To bring it into an abstract Frequency to be recreated in a new pattern outside of something previously created.

You are the most powerful Technology there is. Source Intelligence within you is running a software system that is 100% accurate! If you search outside yourself for an answer, you remain bound in the Matrix. You can't use your outside reality to shift your inside reality! You must choose to move into the Intelligence outside of programming, consciously connect and read information from there without allowing the ego to get in the way!

When you use Evolution Technology, you shift reality. When experiencing the Technology, notice what is happening in your body. Read the patterns by tuning into the sensations! Allow yourself to feel, experience, and witness what you are attaching to within the looping cycle of the Matrix. Observe the energy pattern unfolding.

You are energy and you can obtain information from your body, very much like reading a book. Practice reading energy without becoming the energy or absorbing the energy into your system. This takes Consciousness and practice! Practice reading the Matrix as a way of life! This is how you **"Gamify Reality!"**

You are moving from seeing your body as a reflection of Consciousness to attuning to the body and listening to Consciousness outside of looping patterns, the automatic behaviors of the body. Make this your practice as you ascend.

Your body is not who you are! Your body holds the level of Consciousness that you're able to hold. You begin to bridge from the 3rd to the 4th Body by listening to the Intelligence of your body, the part of your DNA beyond automatic behaviors.

Connect! Practice! Experience! Observe your energy pattern. What happens when you replace an energy pattern with a higher vibrational one? What information or patterns do you discover? Bring in the **Lu, Sca** and **33**. What shifts now?

Learning to identify energy patterns is a superpower. When using Evolution Technology, you attune Consciousness to trace energy patterns. Trust that you are discovering what you need to see. You will always be shown attachments to the looping cycle of the Matrix. When you use Evolution Technology, all that is connected to the looping pattern or program will be removed.

Practice Living From the 4th Level of Consciousness:

Pay attention to where you live life from. Allow yourself to connect to the Intelligence within yourself in order to read information. If you find yourself in the illusion, use the **Lu, Sca** and **33** to shift out of the looping cycle. Allow the shift to happen without letting your will or thoughts get in the way. Are you trying to make it happen or are you allowing the Intelligence to do the work for you?

Spend some time recognizing what level of Consciousness you are expressing. Here is an exercise to demonstrate the difference between allowing the Intelligence to do the work and trying to make it happen.

Exercise:

Shut your eyes and center yourself in your heart space. Take a few deep breaths and clear your mind of any thoughts or worries. Take a moment to feel your connection to the Divine, to Source Frequency.

Now, in your mind's eye, create an image of a sunflower. Observe what the flower looks like and notice what your body is feeling as you bring up the image. Clear your mind of the image.

Return to your heart space and reconnect to Source Frequency. Take a deep breath. Now, ask to be shown an image of a Sunflower. Let the Sunflower create itself. Notice if the image changed. Notice if your body feels different. Is it open and holding a higher Frequency than when you created the image yourself?

Take a moment to reflect on the difference. The first image is created from the 3rd Level of Consciousness. The second image is created from the 4th Level. Your goal is to live more and more of your life in the 4th Level of Consciousness.

Creating the Ascended Human Form

It is time to journey into the magic of creating the Ascended Human Form. The next few chapters will give you support, through very specific exercises, reflections and information, to shift from a body held in the looping cycle of primal programming to becoming 100% Human Potential.

The first part of the journey is to clear the inversion of the chakra system. What does that mean? The chakras are attached to programmed reality. They currently reflect or absorb the energy of the body. They are a hologram of the body. Because the body is held in programmed reality, the chakra system needs to **"turn inside out."** To hold the mastery of the 9, or God Sphere! Doing the exercises below will begin to bring the chakra system into one Frequency of 963 Hz.

It is recommended to do each activation for three days before moving on to the next. During the week, use Consciousness to explore what is changing in your body, your reality and your way of thinking. The more you are conscious of the shift, the more empowering it will be.

Jewels' Story:

"These activations were given to me back in 2015 by a dear friend of mine, Rob Carter, who had passed away. I received them over a period of time, and they were a big part of my first book, <u>Transcendence, A Journey into Oneness through the God Particle</u>. The God Particle is referenced throughout the activations. It is the ability to hold ascended form in Pure Source Frequency and represents an Intelligence beyond the Matrix. Simply said, the God Particle is DMT™, or Source Intelligence, held in a bridge between form and Spirit. It holds the ability to be both in the Frequency of 963 Hz. It is your tuning fork. In some ways, it represents what you are becoming. The God Particle holds Codes that support your Ascension and represents 100% Human Potential."

The chakra system within the Matrix, or programmed reality, creates patterns in a looping cycle stored in energy bodies. This creates both energetic and biological conditions that have been passed down generationally through agreements. These agreements hold information created through reflection of a programmed reality. In essence, the chakra system is unconsciously recreating reincarnation or looping in the life and death cycle, based on basic primitive responses in observation of the Matrix.

As you clear the body of looping cycles, you break repeated patterning and awaken an Intelligence that shifts the chakra system out of primal behavior. You turn the energy body "inside out" and move into expression of Source Intelligence. When this occurs, Source Frequency creates a grid or energetic field for that Intelligence to move online. This allows the body to identify as Frequency without reflection. It breaks the looping cycle of the chakra system and opens the gateway to becoming 100% human potential.

Notes

Notes

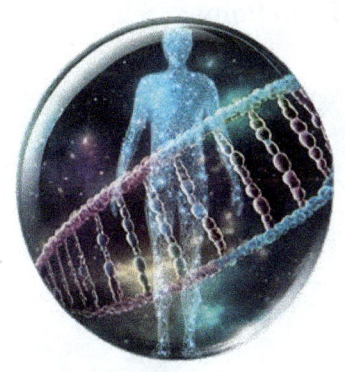

Chapter 11: Awakening The Quantum System: Upgrading The Chakra System To Support The Quantum Body

Meditations of Chakra system 1-9

The Unichio Point holds a gateway to opening up the Pineal Gland. As it opens, it releases DMT™, or the Frequency of 963 Hz. This Frequency holds the Intelligence of Source or the Creator. When turning on the Unichio Point, you support the body to hold this Frequency and prepare it to let go of the need to see itself as energy within the chakra system.

This allows you to move past Ascension symptoms and release old patterns or density held in your energy bodies. Simply put, the Unichio Point puts the body into a reset and allows you to activate the Quantum Body with less stress on your mind, body and spirit.

Activation of the Unichio Point

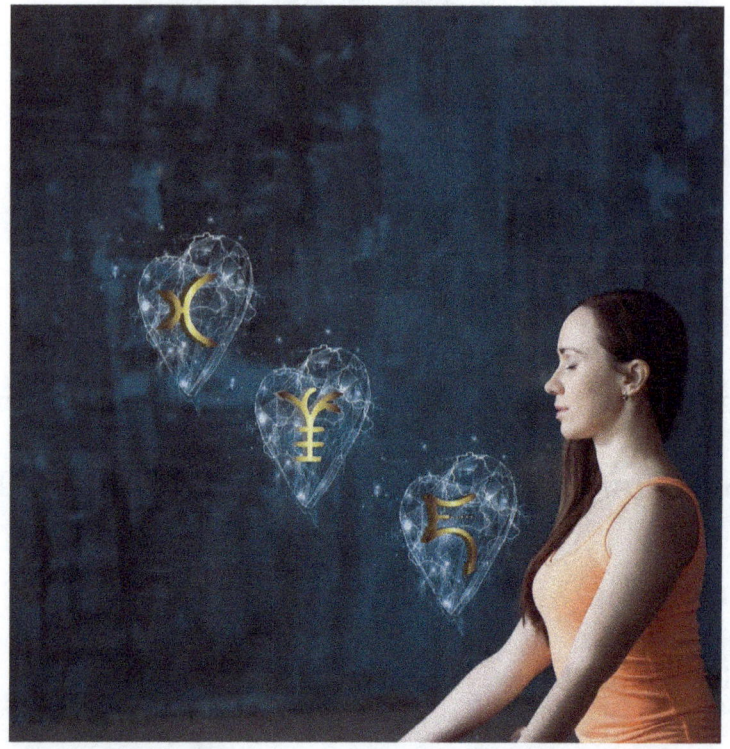

Relax the mind and the body. Let go. Breathe in through the Heart and out through the Heart. Breathe in through the Heart and out through the Heart. Imagine a Pyramid in the center of your Heart. Continue to breathe in and out.

Above you, through space and time, you see the Light of Source. Within this Light is a Hydrogen Atom. This powerful Hydrogen Atom falls down through the stars, through the galaxies and continues to float down into the center of the Pyramid within your Heart. Repeat: **"I ask that the Atom start to spin the Pyramid to the appropriate speed."** You feel the Pyramid start to spin. You feel the power of this Atom within your Pyramid.

With your mind's eye, you go back in time. You travel back as far as you can until you enter the Darkness. Within the Darkness you see a speck of energy. This is Source Intelligence held in the Ascended Particle, the God Particle. You take this Particle and place it in the middle of the Hydrogen Atom. This Pyramid within your Heart is now activated.

See a golden rope of Light flow up to the Pineal Gland from your Heart. Place a beautiful Pyramid in the center. See the Hydrogen Atom within the Light of Source flow down through the top of the Pyramid to the center of the Pineal Gland. Repeat: **"I ask that the Hydrogen Atom spin the Pyramid to the appropriate speed."**

Travel into the Darkness and place the God Particle into the center of the Hydrogen Atom. This activates the Pyramid of the Pineal Gland. The golden rope brings you to the Zeal Point, which is at the base of the skull, where the neck and the skull meet. You place a beautiful Pyramid in the Zeal Point. The Light of Source releases a Hydrogen Atom that flows down to the center of the Pyramid. Repeat: **"I ask that the Hydrogen Atom spin the Pyramid to the appropriate speed."** Now, go into the Darkness and place the God Particle in the center of the Hydrogen Atom within the Pyramid. The Zeal Point is now activated.

All the Pyramids continue to spin at the appropriate speed. Feel the power of these Pyramids. Feel your body rise in vibration as you bring in the knowledge of the Void. The golden rope goes straight forward past the chin, flowing just outside the emotional body about two feet. This is the Unichio Point.

This is the chakra that opens to Christ Consciousness. You see a beautiful Pyramid placed in the middle of the Unichio Point. The Light of Source releases a very powerful Hydrogen Atom and places it in the center of the Pyramid. Repeat: **"I ask for the Pyramid of my Unichio point to spin at the appropriate speed."**

Traveling into the Darkness, you place the God Particle in the center of the Hydrogen Atom. The Unichio Point is now activated, connecting to Christ Consciousness. The Unichio Point follows along the golden rope until it rests in the middle of the throat. The Zeal Point meets the Unichio Point in the throat, forming a Pyramid on top of a Pyramid, a Merkabah. The atoms and the God Particles meet and become one powerful energy. The Merkabah spins at the appropriate speed.

The Pyramid of your Heart follows the golden rope up to the Pyramid of the Pineal Gland. As these Pyramids meet, they form a Merkabah. The Hydrogen Atoms and God Particles merge, becoming one energy. The Merkabah begins to spin at the appropriate speed. The Merkabah in the throat flows up inside the Merkabah within the Pineal Gland. The Merkabahs join together as a twelve-pointed star.

The Hydrogen Atoms and God Particles become one, spinning at the appropriate speed. This twelve-pointed star, a Merkabah inside of a Merkabah, flows down along the golden rope back to your Heart Chakra, becoming one. This programs the Heart into Christ Consciousness, activating the Template of the Trinity. Repeat: **"Thank you. It is done."**

Do the next activations and wait three to four days before moving on. Even better, do one every day for a week and explore the Consciousness or Intelligence that shifts you out of the programmed body into the Quantum Body. Use your intuition to explore. Note the Level of Consciousness you are exploring from.

Activation 1 Chakras 1-4: Root Chakra to the Heart Chakra

Breathe in through the Heart and out through the Heart. Breathe in through the Heart and out through the Heart. Experience your body as the Quantum Grid. Feel the Quantum reality in every cell and every molecule within your DNA and all your energy systems. Your body is a creation of Source Intelligence. Feel yourself vibrate with the Frequency held here.

A Hydrogen Atom enters your Root Chakra. At the very center is the Flower of Life that contains the God Particle. The Hydrogen Atom easily migrates into the center of the God Particle, just like a key enters a keyhole, and clicks once to the right. As the Hydrogen Atom clicks within the God Particle, the Flower begins to spin.

Feel your frequency rise. When the Frequency of 111 Hz. is reached, the Flower collapses within the God Particle, creating a gateway through the Void and into the Sacral Chakra.

The Hydrogen Atom flows up through this gateway and into the Flower held there. In the center of the Flower is the God Particle. The Hydrogen Atom flows up from the Earth into the God Particle, clicking once to the right. The Flower begins to spin and as it reaches the Frequency of 222 Hz., the Flower collapses into the God Particle, creating a gateway within the Void between the Sacral Chakra and the Solar Plexus. These Frequencies bring in the vibration of Oneness. Feel the vibration enter every cell and every molecule of your body.

The Hydrogen Atom raises up through this gateway, through the Void, into the Solar Plexus. See the Flower within the Solar Plexus as the Hydrogen Atom easily flows from the Earth into the center of the God

Particle, clicking once to the right. The Flower begins to spin. Feel the spin creating the Frequency of 333 Hz. When the Flower reaches the frequency of 333 Hz., it collapses into the center of the God Particle, creating a gateway into the Void between the Solar Plexus and the Heart.

Experience the Frequency of your body rising even higher. Feel the Frequencies move into all the energy centers, into every cell and molecule. The Hydrogen Atom raises up through the gateway of your Solar Plexus into your Heart Chakra. The Hydrogen Atom flows from the Earth into the Flower. It enters the God Particle, clicks once to the right and allows it to spin. The spin accelerates to the Frequency of 444 Hz. As the spin reaches the Frequency of 444 Hz., the Flower collapses into the God Particle, creating a beautiful golden Pyramid.

All these Frequencies are held within the Pyramid. The Heart Pyramid holds the Flower of Life. The Flower transcends time and space. Transcends judgment and separation. You are now vibrating in the Frequency of Love. Allow the Frequency to take over your body, transforming the cells and DNA with the knowledge held within the Flower of Life. Repeat: **"Thank you. It is done."**

Reflection:

Your lower brain is fighting to survive. The ego is connected to fight or flight. It strives to create in order to keep itself alive. The ego survives through separation, knowing that if the mind of the Soul were to activate completely, the ego would no longer exist. The ego uses every trick to keep you stuck in the only reality it knows, creating separation. The ego holds onto 3rd dimension programming connected to survival.

All living things live in the program of survival: animals, plants and you. Your entire life is programmed to "survive" over all else. This is the illusion of the 3rd dimension. It is time to break the illusion of death. Death of the physical body! Death of the ego! They are one and the same. For the ego to die, and for you to live in the Quantum Body, is to live outside the boundaries of death. The ego cannot survive in this reality.

Allow the lower brain to lose its programming by identifying its control over you. Next time you are "thinking," notice what you need. You will know what part of the brain you are in by the way your Heart feels. If your thoughts are connected to the ego, programmed in fight or flight, you will feel contracted and ready for action. Notice the energy trying to create a reality with your thoughts. Your ego wants you to create from the lower brain to make you "safe" in the world, to "survive" in order to exist. To create from ego is to create from fear and separation.

When you are connected to the Intelligence of the Quantum Body, you will feel an open Heart. You may hear your ego in the background attempting to pull you back in. The mind of the Soul allows the Frequency of 963 Hz. to bring in thoughts and experiences from a new reality created from the Intelligence of Source. The more you listen to the programming of Divine Mind, the stronger it becomes and the more your reality shifts into the Quantum Field. You create as Source. This is the Quantum Life. This brings all creation into Oneness.

The programming of the lower mind is dying. The ego will desperately try to hold onto this reality by bringing up all your primal fears and survival patterns. It's not the truth. Identify the game and decide it is not the way you want to play anymore. In time, Source Intelligence stored in the DNA will become your state of being. You will no longer exist in the identity of the ego. You will rest in the stillness of the Mind of the Creator. It is then that you will be "all that is" in the Frequency of Oneness.

Activation 2: Chakras 5-9

Bring your attention to the Trinity of your Heart. Invite the programmed mind and body to meet in the gateway of your Heart. At the center of the gateway is the God Particle. Beams of Light connect to the points of the Trinity created through the mind, body and spirit. A beam of silver, gold and purple shines to the corners. The colors bring in love, peace and bliss, flowing through your Heart and connecting to crystalline formations in the core of the physical body.

The energy then connects to your mind, the programmed responses of your brain. Your body holds the gateway to the Quantum Field beyond observation. See energetic roots extend from your High Heart into the core of the Earth. Allow the roots to reach the stars above. You connect to "all that is" as the Trinity begins to spin.

The Trinity, mind, body and spirit, enters the God Particle, moving into the Darkness, the Void. The energies of the Trinity merge with Source Intelligence, bringing power, knowledge and wisdom into One. As the energies attune you to the Quantum Body, the Light enters through the top of your head, flowing down through the spine and connecting with the God Particle in the Heart. This creates a gateway from the Heart Chakra to the Throat Chakra.

From the core of the Earth and the stars above, two Hydrogen Atoms travel through your energy system. Both enter the gateway into the 5th Chakra, where the Flower of Life rests. The Hydrogen Atoms migrate to the center of the Flower, enter the God Particle and click three times to the right. They start at the 9:00 position on a clock and move to the 6:00 position. Next, from the 6:00 position to the 3:00 position. Then, from the 3:00 position to the 12:00 position. They create a full circle in reverse, erasing all time, karma and cosmic law.

As the circle is completed, the Light expands out through all existence, merging all existence within the Light. As it reaches the Frequency of 555 Hz., "all that is" collapses into the God Particle and creates a gateway into the 3rd Eye.

The Hydrogen Atoms of the core of the Earth and the stars enter through the gateway, gravitating to the center of the Flower within the 3rd Eye. Both Hydrogen Atoms migrate into the God Particle, clicking three times to the right, completing the circle and erasing all karma and law. The Light expands out, collecting "all that is," raising the Frequency to 666 Hz. As it reaches the Frequency of 666 Hz., all existence collapses into the Flower of the 3rd Eye. All of existence within the 3rd Eye becomes One with the God Particle, opening the gateway into the Crown Chakra.

The Hydrogen Atoms of the core of the Earth and the Star of Bethlehem enter through this gateway, flowing into the center of the Flower of the Crown. As they enter the God Particle, it creates three clicks to the right, completing the circle. The Light merges with "all that is," raising the Frequency to 777 Hz.

As all existence becomes one with the Light, it collapses into the Flower of Life, creating a gateway into the 8th Chakra. The Hydrogen Atoms of the core of the Earth and the stars flow up through this gateway into the 8th Chakra, where the Flower of Life rests. The Hydrogen Atoms migrate to the center of the God Particle, clicking three times to the right, completing the circle, erasing all karma and law. As the circle is completed, the Light expands out, collecting "all that is," bringing in the Frequency of 888 Hz. As the frequency of 888 Hz. is reached, "all that is" collapses into the Flower, creating a gateway into the 9th Chakra.

The Hydrogen Atom of the core of the Earth and the stars flow through this gateway to the center of the Flower. The Atoms enter the God Particle, clicking three times to the right, completing the circle and erasing karma and law. This expands the Light into "all that is," bringing in the Frequency of 963 Hz. As it reaches the Frequency of 963 Hz., all of existence collapses into the God Particle within the Flower of Life. This creates a channel that runs through the Crown Chakra, down the spine and out the Root Chakra. All the colors of Light freely move throughout this channel. It is in this channel that all becomes One, creating the gateway into the Quantum Body.

Reflection:

What Is the Earth Becoming as You Ascend?

Ask for your energetic body to merge with the grid of your Higher Self in the multi-dimensions. Remember you are more than form. You are Quantum. During Ascension, the energy moving through you and your reality is connected to Frequencies holding energetic portals. These allow downloads, or higher Frequencies, to enter the Matrix and activate your dormant DNA codes. An energy charge is created that brings your physical body into your Ascended Body and begins your Ascension, beyond the Matrix itself. Earth's energy grid creates a vortex that expands over the entire world. The grid of your physical body and the Earth body merge and create the Advanced Human Experience.

The awakening of DMT™ transcends and reprograms the energetic genetic coding of all humanity and 3rd dimension reality. You are shedding programming, how the brain, cells and genetics perceive your world and the way you emotionally process information in your experiences. The brain develops new synapse responses and neurotransmitters that respond from DNA Intelligence and no longer operate from the "fight or flight" response in the lower part of the brain. This minimizes fear and allows you to respond with a higher perspective.

DNA expression is in alignment with a solar wave of the Sun which creates a gateway between the Quantum Body and the Advanced Human. Ask to experience DNA Intelligence to connect to the YOU already existing as the Ascended Human. This connects the brain and heart waves of the YOU in this reality through DNA Intelligence and integrates the multi-dimensional waves that are the vehicle into the new reality you are creating.

You are building a grid in the higher Frequencies of the Quantum Field. The Earth opens a new vortex that spreads a grid of energetic responses in the codes of the Earth's Matrix. The Earth contains responses just like the human body. To match the new reality, body systems upgrade simultaneously with the Earth. Humans and the Earth become an energy grid. You become Source Intelligence as the Quantum Field. Together the Quantum Body and the Quantum Earth vibrate to the Frequency beyond the God Sphere or identity in form, transporting all existence into the Frequency of Source Intelligence.

Activation of the Quantum Body: Dissolving the Illusion of the Chakra System and the Inversion of the Tree of Life

Expanding into the Quantum Body, breathe in through the Heart and out through the Heart. Again, breathe in through the Heart and out through the Heart. Connect to the Trinity of the Heart, mind, body and Spirit. Breathe up and down the channel, from the top of your crown to your root. Breathe up and down this channel.

As you breathe, notice a particle of Light in each of the nine Chakras that hold all of existence, the Quantum Field. The channel contains the Light. As you breathe, allow this Light to expand to the front, to the sides, to the back. Allow it to flow through the top of your head and down out the bottom of your feet. Let the Light fill your being and extend about four feet from your body.

The Light contains the energy grid of your Quantum Self existing in the Quantum Field. Allow this grid to merge with your energy system. Each God Particle in the chakras holds a place for the Tree of Life. They begin to migrate to their appropriate spots within and around your body. Your body becomes the Quantum Field.

The Unichio Point begins to spin as it migrates to the God Particle of the Heart. As it enters the Heart, the Frequency of all the other Particles rises to the Frequency of Source. The Unichio Point has brought Source Consciousness into the Heart.

The God Particle of the Root Chakra begins to spin, migrates up the spine, enters the Heart and becomes One. The God Particle of the Sacral Chakra begins to spin and, as it spins, flows through the Tree of Life, enters the Heart and becomes One. The God Particle of the Solar Plexus Chakra begins to spin. As it spins, it flows into the Heart Center and becomes One.

Feel the vibration run through your body as you become closer to the Frequency of Source. Let go of all fear and enter the Darkness. The God Particle of the Throat Chakra begins to spin. It flows down through the spine into the Heart, becoming One. The God Particle of the 3rd Eye Chakra begins to spin. As it spins, it migrates through the sacred channel, the spine, into the Heart Center and becomes One.

Feel yourself resonating with the God Particle as you become One with "all that is." The Particle of the Crown Chakra begins to spin. As it spins, it migrates down through the Tree of Life into the Center of the Heart and becomes One. The God Particle of the 8th Chakra begins to spin. As it spins, it flows into the Heart Center, becoming One. The God Particle of the 9th Chakra begins to spin. As it spins, it travels down through the spine and enters the Heart Center, becoming One.

All the Particles exist as one energy within the Heart. The Heart opens and expands. The First Particle of Existence begins to spin. As it spins, it flows through the spine and enters the Heart Center. The vibration of the Heart rises into Source Consciousness. The Heart expands into a space just above the physical heart, creating your Sacred Heart. The Sacred Heart begins to spin, absorbing "all that is:" the Light, your energy grid, your energy body and your physical body. Everything enters the Sacred Heart. All become One within the God Particle. Allow the Frequency to resonate within you. Be still and know you are the Creator; you are the Quantum Field.

Notes

Notes

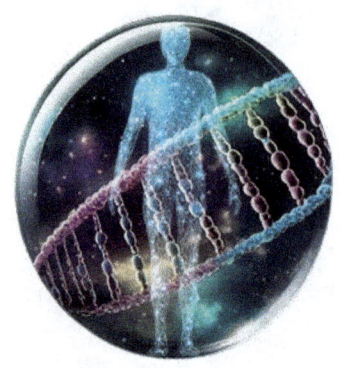

Chapter 12: Breaking the God Code: The Inversion of the Cells

Within the programmed body, you create and repeat patterns in looping cycles. These have been passed down through your biology. Thus, cells unconsciously recreate the life and death cycle based on basic primitive tissue.

Using Evolution Technology, you break the looping cycle of repeated cellular patterning and awaken an Intelligence that shifts cells out of primal behavior into direct expression of Source Intelligence. The cells shift away from holding and expressing information from their environment.

A complex system or energetic field is created wherein Source Intelligence moves online. This allows the body to identify as Frequency without reflection and breaks the looping cycle of cellular behavior. You see beyond illusion! You master the Matrix! Human potential evolves to 100% expression of Source Intelligence and you **"Break the God Code!"**

Using Evolution Technology, cells become a direct reflection of the God Sphere. You activate DNA Frequencies to shift cells into expression of Source Intelligence beyond the Sphere all together.

What Are Epigenetics and How Can We Turn Them Off?

Epigenetics is the study of changes in organisms caused by modification of gene expression rather than alteration of the genetic code itself. Epigenetic codes get "turned on" by the environment in which the cell exists. Diet, thoughts and beliefs, toxins and the collective reality you agree to, both consciously and unconsciously, create the environment of your body.

Epigenetics are codes that move into expression when the frequency of the environment is sustained long enough to signal the cell, your DNA, to turn on that expression. This alters the cell to duplicate in the expression of the code that is turned on. Aging is an epigenetic code. It is a collective agreement that, over time, you age. There is no biological reason to age.

The great thing about epigenetic codes is that, because you are not born with them "turned on," they can be "turned off" by changing the environment of the cells. You change the cell to change the environment. You shift the Frequency of the cell by clearing out low vibrational beliefs and agreements that keep the cell in a looping cycle of age and disease.

Presently, you identify within your environment. You see what has been created or proven and agree as a collective or as an individual that it is true. Most often, you do this without even questioning it!

As an Advanced Conscious Being, you can turn this "inside out." You can shift the reality of the cell by giving it an identity, an "I AM statement", to hold while moving the cell into expression of the new identity. The cell no longer looks outside itself to be told what to do. It becomes the expression of a higher Frequency and no longer unconsciously agrees with the environment within which it has existed. Your cell becomes conscious!

I AM…

I AM Responsible For My Own Life.
I AM Limitless.
I AM Love.
I AM The CEO Of My Body.
I AM Happy.
I AM Magical And Make The Impossible, Possible.
I AM Wealthy.
I AM A Divine Miracle.
I AM Creative.
I AM Aligned With Divine Will.
I AM Joy.
I AM Capable.
I AM Abundant.
I AM Safe And Secure.
I AM A Wonderful Wife/Husband, Etc.
I AM Supported.
I AM A Caring Person.
I AM Nourished With Divine Love.
I AM A Money Magnet.
I AM Filled With Vitality.
I AM Valuable.

I AM The Joy Of Life, Expressing & Receiving.
I AM Loveable.
I AM Peace, Love And Joy.
I AM Terrific.
I AM A Caring Person.
I AM Healthy.
I AM The Light Of Transformation In The World.
I AM Positive.
I AM Wealthy, So Others Can Be Too.
I AM Inspiring.
I AM FreeTo Be Who I Want To Be.
I AM Resourceful.
I AM Free To Express My Truth & Light In The World.
I AM Eternal.
I AM Loved Unconditionally.
I AM Radiant.
I AM The Master Of My Own Life.
I AM Successful.
I AM United And Whole.
I AM Beautiful.
I AM One With The Divine.
I AM A Channel OF Divine Grace.
I AM Solid In My Power And Who I AM.
I AM Blessed.
I AM A Divine Gift To This World.
I AM Grateful.
I AM Owning My Divine Sovereign Power & Right.
I AM Powerful.
I AM The Authority Of My Life.
I AM Divine.

I AM The Master Of My Body.

I AM Free To Be Me.

I AM Successful In All I Do.

I AM Strong.

I AM In Divine Flow.

I AM Light.

I AM Divine Creation And Celebrate Who I Am.

I AM The Way.

I AM Here To Be An Expression of The Divine.

I AM Truth.

I AM Infused With Divine Light & Consciousness.

I AM Connected To My Soul.

I AM Divine Perfection.

I AM Prosperous And Abundance Comes To Me Easily.

I AM Accepting The Perfection Of Who I Am.

I AM The Most Amazing Treasure In The Universe.

I AM At Peace With My Life/Body.

Likely, you see the body, or the part of you that is conscious of yourself as a body, as separate from the mind. Science is now showing that your organs and cells have Consciousness.

The truth is your body is your Consciousness! The more you reprogram your cells to awaken to Source Intelligence stored in the DNA, the more you, as the conscious observer, meet this Intelligence with awareness. You also awaken to potential beyond programmed reality. This is the evolution of mankind!

The more you "turn on" Codes that express Source Intelligence that lay dormant in the DNA, the more you shift what it is to be human. You use only 10-12% of your capabilities in the programmed reality you have agreed to. When you consciously reprogram your cells to shift in identity/Frequency from what you have agreed to, you move past programming and into creation of what is beyond what has already been created.

The Process of Moving from Collective Consciousness into Higher Consciousness:

Separating from the ego and choosing a higher Consciousness allows you to observe yourself. Judging what is being observed is an indication that ego has taken over. Mental chatter reflects fear of letting go, the need to control a situation or the need to process.

Processing is questioning what the ego is saying. The ego holds thoughts connected to duality from social consciousness. It is the story of humanity. Breaking free of thought forms is a process. To do this, you must identify with the situation/story by questioning yourself.

First, ask:
- **Do my thoughts have a purpose?**
- **Are my thoughts giving me information?**
- **Is there a new vibration around my thoughts that wasn't there before?**
- **Am I cycling the "same old story" that keeps going around and around in my head?**

After identifying the story that is playing out, you may want to visit this next set of questions to proceed with your clearing. Write down your answers and feelings during this time.

- What did I discover that is causing me stress?
- Can I remove duality?
- What do I need?
- Am I looking for validation?
- Do I need someone on my side?
- Am I needing the situation to "fit" my idea of what I feel is right or just?

If you are looking for justification, validation, or a desire for someone to take your side, you are coming from ego. Congratulations! Identifying "'the story" is the first step to becoming the observer. The ego is now being observed instead of running the show.

Ask yourself:

- Is this situation worth losing energy over?
- Is it important that I win in order to feel like I'm getting what I want? Is winning how I wish to receive energy?
- What is this experience teaching me?
- How can I remain neutral?
- Am I trying to control the outcome to feel safe?
- Am I afraid of what others will think if I don't "do something?"

Listen to inner guidance and allow a shift from ego to stillness. Allow others to have their experience without needing to be right or wrong. Hold space that neither person nor opinion needs to be agreed with for you to have your own experience, regardless of what your ego is saying in the background. Hold the situation in Love.

Allow yourself to create an outcome without expectation. This invites the Intelligence to take over. When you view a situation through Source Intelligence, the world becomes magical. All interactions become information the Intelligence is offering you; you interact with that information as the Intelligence itself. Thus, allowing the programmed mind to dissolve and you to experience the Quantum Body as Source Intelligence.

Clearing Duality Meditation:

The purpose of this meditation is to clear duality and bring all existence into Oneness by connecting to the Quantum Body. See a beautiful iridescent gold Pyramid, with violet at the top, silver at the right corner and white at the left corner. All parts are iridescent and vibrate at 963 Hz. The energies of the body and mind meet in the center of the Pyramid.

See your body as a grid. Within the grid, you release programs that keep you in duality. The Light streams down through the channel that runs along your spine. The Light absorbs the synapse and neurotransmitter responses within the brain and heart that keep you stuck in duality. As these programs are absorbed, they leave space, which becomes an empty Void within you. The Void holds Source Intelligence, no thought, no memory. Just be in the Now moment as Source Frequency.

The Light expands out within the channel of your spine. It expands out in all directions, fills your aura and absorbs all energetic blocks, programs and frequencies connected to duality. Feel space within the Light. Feel the Frequency of Source.

Before you, you see a Veil. This is the Veil that keeps you separate from all that is. Through the Veil you see a glimpse of yourself as the Advanced Human. Walk towards the Veil as the Light merges fully with your body. You are cleared of all frequencies held in duality as you easily walk through the Veil. You feel your vibration rise. You become one with the Quantum Field as it awakens within the Trinity of your Heart. Allow the Trinity to spin. As it spins, It brings the mind, body and spirit into the Frequency of 963 Hz.

The gateway of your heart opens to the Quantum Field. The Trinity is absorbed into Source Frequency. The Frequency of Source absorbs all that exists within your identity, creating Zero Point. As you journey through the Quantum Field, all of evolution is reprogrammed to the Frequency of Source. Everything that was once observed holds the Frequency of 963 Hz.

This is your Quantum Body. You feel no separation. You feel no fear. You see life through the Intelligence of Source. Your body glows with the Light of Source. You know that you exist in the Quantum Field. Your journey becomes one of evolution into the Advanced Human. Allow your body to absorb this new Frequency. Allow the new synapse responses of the brain and heart to reprogram to hold the Frequency of 963 Hz. You have awakened your Quantum Body. You are living within the Intelligence of Source.

Notes

Notes

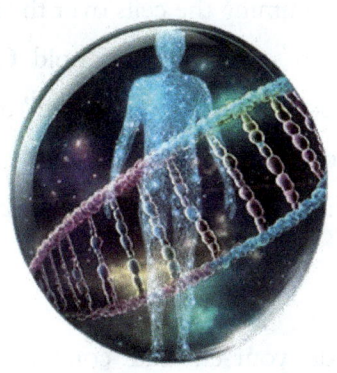

Chapter 13: Creating the Quantum Body

When you focus on reprogramming the mind, you reprogram only 10% of the electrons of the body. Electrons hold Consciousness. The mind is hardwired to receive information through observation, creating the loop of the body's experience of age and disease. The cells of the body function within this loop since Consciousness is currently held through the experience of programmed reality. The environment of the cells is created by the Level of Consciousness being held. If Consciousness is held through observation, a loop is created, and the cells of the body will also loop, thus creating the life and death cycle.

When you activate Source Codes within the DNA and allow Consciousness to identify in the Frequency of these Codes, the Electrons of the cells observe this Intelligence instead of the environment of the body or programmed mind. This activates Consciousness in the other 90% of the body. The Electrons awaken Consciousness connected to Source Intelligence through DNA expression.

With this shift, reprogramming the cells over the mind, you activate the other 90% of the body's electricity to hold Consciousness beyond programmed reality. Consciousness "turns on" through Source Codes, bypassing observation of the Matrix. The body is the most advanced Technology of anything created in the Matrix. The body is pure Source Intelligence.

When you go outside yourself and connect to the frequency of information there, you reconnect to the Matrix. Unless experienced through the Intelligence of Source in expression, it's the Matrix.

You have the ability to use reflection to see programmed reality. You can then access Source Intelligence beyond what is seen. Imagine it like turning on a Frequency of information from Source that is 100% accurate. Then use Consciousness to attune to what the information is saying. Once you have the information, move into expression of that information beyond observing it. This allows you to go from the 3rd to the 4th and finally to the 5th Level of Consciousness.

The first step to break the body's looping cycle of age and disease is to begin playing as the Creator of the Matrix itself. There's nothing "wrong" with the Matrix; it is a complete looping system. The brilliance behind the Matrix is its Consciousness. It is the creator of the game in which you choose to play. It's here to help you exit out of it.

Learn to use the Consciousness of your body in the Matrix. Its intelligence is very slow moving but is here to support you in shifting to the Quantum Body. If you have pain or something going on in your body, it's the body's way of showing you density. That the particles are going really slow because they're in degeneration. Instead of pointing out all of what you perceive to be "flaws," see each as Consciousness giving you a stairway to your next higher Frequency. Realize that the body is just giving you information. It's still embedded in the Matrix but offers you a way to tap into a higher level of Consciousness that shares what to do next. You will always receive answers. The Matrix will always loop in front of you as to what it wants you to pay attention to. There's always a Higher Intelligence trying to bridge information to you.

In the 2nd Body, the body is a direct reflection of Consciousness. When working with the 2nd Body and your most dominant energy, any dense information that repeatedly gets your attention, creates a bridge to Source Intelligence. Connect to the Frequency of the ascended state of that which you are wanting to shift. Ask it to activate that specific DNA Code. Use your body as Consciousness. Affirm an intention that you are creating a bridge to understand the Intelligence coming through. Even if it doesn't show itself right away, put the bridge there so as to invite the information to come forth.

Source Intelligence is always available to tap into. It's right there but your Consciousness may not have caught up yet to feel it, see it, be it. The easy way to do this is the 1 to the 2 to the 3 to the 1. (See next page.) The bridge is the ability to see what's there and link you into the Frequency of that Intelligence (3) beyond the loop itself. The bridge is the awareness that you are always in the illusion. Until you become 100% Source Intelligence, you will attune to the Intelligence with the Level of Consciousness you are holding. Keep going! There is always something beyond what you now understand.

1-2-3-1 Method:

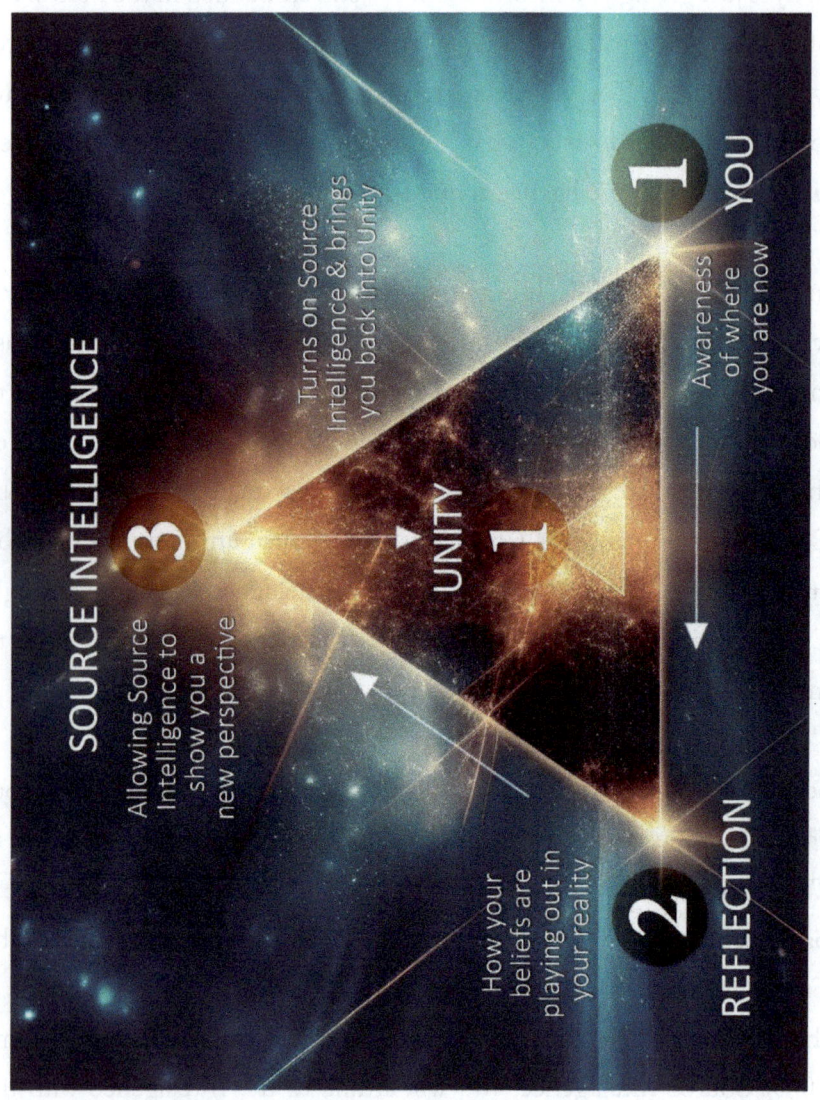

https://becomingbioquantum.com/1-2-3-1

The Matrix is brilliant as to how it catapults you to real information. Know that you have this awareness. The body talks to you in so many ways. Notice that the parts of your life you resist show up frequently in looping patterns. Start bridging these experiences into Source Intelligence by using the tools given in this book.

Dominant body awareness, such as pain or wrinkles, has Consciousness and has information. You can meet each at the level of Consciousness it's holding in that slower spin state or create a bridge to the information beyond it. Because you are conscious that this state exists, it will reflect back to you that level of Consciousness.

But you have the ability to create a bridge to Source Intelligence to where lower dense forms, that are plugged into the looping cycle, have the ability to move up in Frequency to create a new experience. This means you can create a faster spin state where density is released, and the Consciousness of the experience moves up. You are able to meet it in a Frequency consciously in a new state, a faster spin rate from beyond space and time. Thus, you master the 2nd Body!

You repeat this over and over, using Consciousness through the experience of Source Intelligence until you become Source Intelligence. Because you are still naming the body, you use the ability to name what's happening in the body to ascend the Consciousness it's holding.

The body already knows it's whole. It knows its original Divine Blueprint. It knows how to self-heal. Use the reflection of the Matrix and the body to become the NEXT in human evolution.

Consciousness gives you a stairway to the next state of Consciousness. The body knows this. The Quantum Body knows it's perfect, that there's nothing to heal, that it's resetting to its original blueprint. The only reason you experience the need to heal is that you identify in a frequency of a lower spin state, the programmed body.

The bridge makes it easier to move into a Frequency Pattern that's beyond what the experience of Consciousness is. The 2nd Body is very powerful, and you will return to it even as you sit in the 3rd Body. You will consistently use the 2nd Body to be able to shift to the 3rd.

As you begin to activate your Divine Technology by awakening DNA Intelligence, language will change. Communication through the universal language will be the next step in delivering specific Frequencies as you shift into the Light Body. You can use holographic imaging to see through the illusion of both form and programming of words. This allows you to be everything and nothing at the same time. The vehicle, particle Light form, connects to the grid turning on DMT™ codes.

Are you ready to BREAK the looping cycle of the body? To open the pathway into existing outside of the Matrix? To break the God Code? The Quantum Body holds the Intelligence of what you are becoming. This level of Intelligence has no Consciousness, meaning it has no need to be conscious of itself because it holds the Intelligence of all things without the need for reflection. Just sit with this.

This is going to be a WILD RIDE! Buckle up! Reality is bending. What if everything you know to be true isn't true?

The Equation of the Ascended Body: Breaking the Matrix

The Electrons of the Quantum Body are not negative or positive, are not an element and are not in form. Electrons hold a Frequency which can be used to create a pattern of Intelligence within the Quantum Body. Electrons hold your Consciousness. Your body is the

Intelligence, so the body has something to see itself as while it shifts from form to identifying as Frequency.

When the Electrons connect to DMT™, Source Intelligence, the body runs Frequency Patterns just like a circuit. It is able to run millions of circuits, each giving different information in Frequency from Source Intelligence. The Electrons ascend into the Quantum Body and create a gateway for the body to identify from form to Frequency through an organic grid system or Divine Technology. The grid system holds Intelligence in a Frequency as Consciousness shifts from identifying in the primal body to the Quantum Body.

Electrons play a significant role in becoming the Quantum Body, the Advanced Human. As you break through the Matrix, the Quantum Body activates an organic Technology to move you out of the illusion of the programmed body and attunes your Consciousness to what you are becoming. Electrons "exist without existing" in Consciousness but hold Consciousness in expression, meaning they are conscious beyond observation of their reality.

Electrons build in the body as you shift from density to higher spin states. The DNA holds the core memory of Source Intelligence. As the body turns on Codes of memory, the cell structure shifts to a higher Frequency. Over time, as the body holds higher Frequencies, it begins to move from density to waves or Ascended Light. Conscious awareness of the shift facilitates thought through core memory. First, your body realizes the shift is happening, allowing you to consciously follow.

Evolution of the body occurs when DMT™ Frequency moves into the Electrons of the body. This brings the cells into a high spin rate while connecting to a system of Frequency held in Source Intelligence, the Quantum Body.

When conscious thought meets Source Intelligence held in DMT™, you move into vehicles of energy, Source Expression. This Expression is held outside universal laws or the looping cycles held in density. The Ascended Body can only be fully expressed when reflection of information or reality is diminished. The Ascended Body cannot be achieved through the illusion of the Matrix. The Matrix must be experienced through the Technology activated through DMT™, Electrons and the Intelligence held in the DNA.

When activating specific coding in the DNA, a vibration moves through the looping cycles of the body and turns on Source Intelligence. When this happens, you consciously experience different levels of identity within the Frequencies, affecting both body and mind. It may seem as though you move beyond time and space yet remain anchored in the 3rd dimension. It is as if you have a foot in two worlds. This will be your experience until full expression of the Source Template is achieved.

You can use your reality as information by reading lower frequencies as they come into your field of reference. When in this awareness, lower frequencies become neutralized, allowing higher Frequency realities to appear. Allow yourself to enjoy the miracles of higher Frequencies that hold Source Intelligence beyond the sensation of density.

Mastering this experience will be another step to moving into the Quantum Body. A supernatural existence bends the holographic grid, the Matrix, held in lower frequency patterns. You will provide a huge service to humanity and all beings stuck in the time space continuum/looping cycle. It is time to **Break the Matrix!**

Knowing what Level of Consciousness your body is holding is a huge part of surrendering to DMT™ Intelligence. The 1st Level of Consciousness is the awareness that you are more than your body. The 2nd Level of Consciousness is that your body is a direct reflection of Consciousness. If you remain in that space, you do not break the looping cycle.

When you gain awareness that you are naming the experience of your body, you have the opportunity to move beyond the body. In the looping cycle, thought leads the body. When you have awareness that Consciousness is a direct reflection of the body, you hold the body at that level of Consciousness. In the Quantum Body, you turn on DMT™ Intelligence in the DNA. You move into a Frequency where the body leads to what you consider to be thought. Thought then moves behind the body.

Think of it like this. Consciousness always follows the Intelligence of your Quantum Body. In the beginning you will attune Consciousness to the body so the body can tell you what it needs in order to move into the Quantum Field.

If you continue to do everything from your thoughts, thinking that the body will follow, you will not break out of the looping cycle. You must master the 2nd Ascended Body or your thoughts will always be leading the body. And the body will not have the chance to show you that it knows more than you do.

Practice putting your thoughts behind the body. Attune to what the body is telling you and let it lead. Remember, your Quantum Body is the most advanced Technology there is. Let it show you just how powerful you are beyond the limitation of your mind.

As you activate your Quantum Body, notice from what Level you are experiencing it. This allows you to choose to move into the 4th or 5th Level of Consciousness and bypass the loop of your programming. Remember, the 3rd Level of Consciousness is "trying to make it happen." It is creating a program from your programming.

Notes

Notes

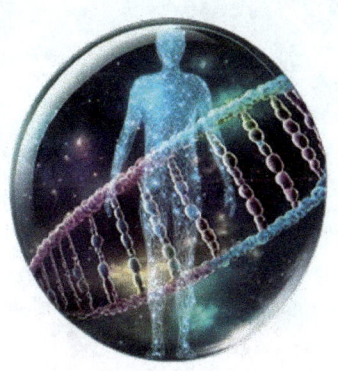

Chapter 14: Consciously Awakening The Quantum Body

1st Level of the Ascended Form (1st Body)

The 1st Ascended Body is the Awakening Level. Your heart has been plugged into a frequency pattern or timeline connected to the Matrix. This creates slow degeneration over time.

The 1st Body also works with the 2nd Element: **"I AM Not My Thoughts"**. The mind is your agreement of how you think of yourself in the Matrix. In this Level of the Ascended Body, you are aware that density is contained in space. You begin to break the illusion that the body is the self, that the experience of the body is who you are.

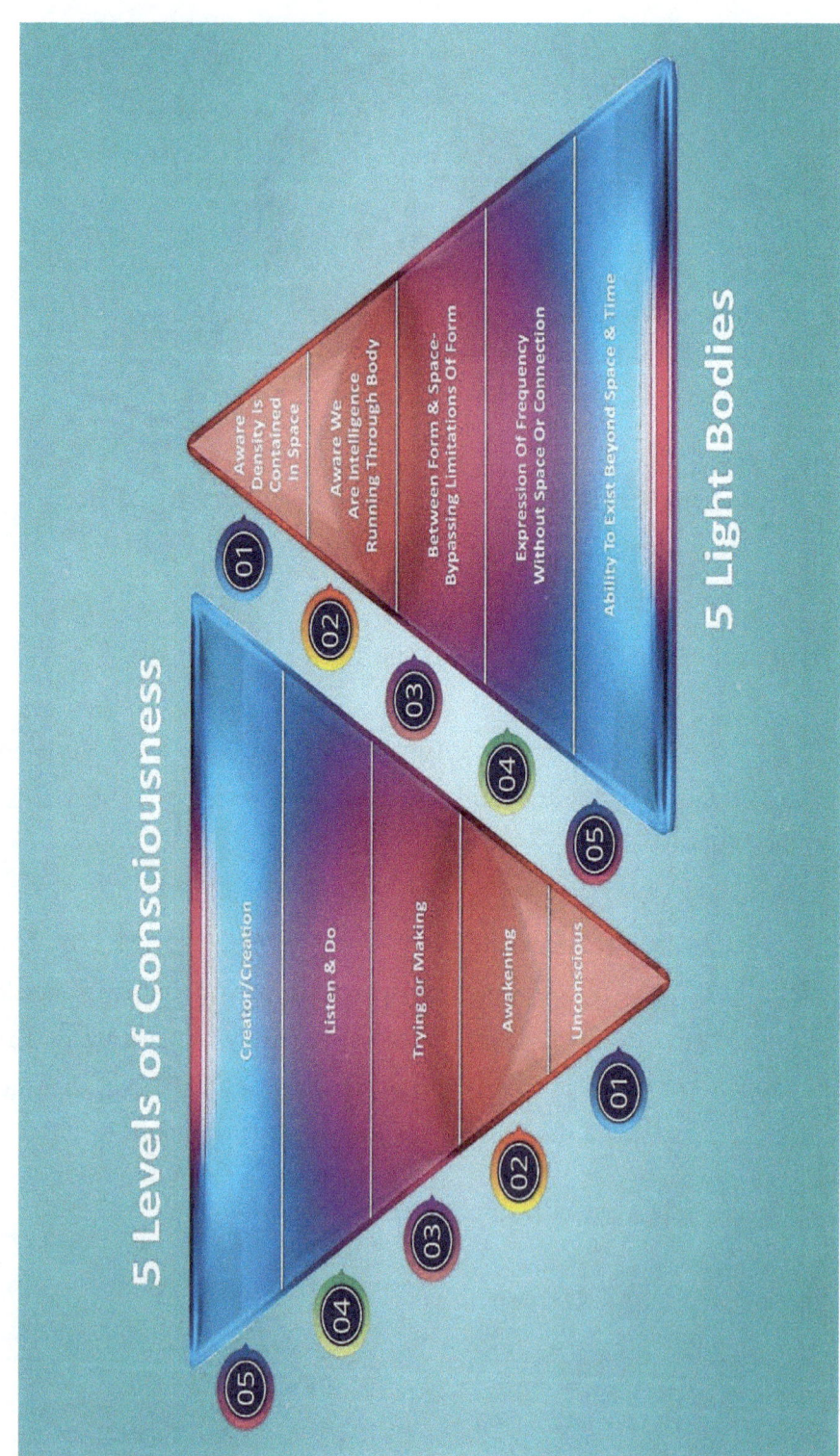

5 Levels of Consciousness connected to 5 Light Bodies

This is the stage where you become aware that you are more than the experience of form. When you realize you are not the body, DNA awakens, and cellular structure begins to shift. This creates space between reality and allows an Intelligence beyond the programming of the body to come forth. The body then "turns on" Frequencies that elevate Consciousness beyond programming.

Exercise:

Use the 3 Symbols of **Lu, Sca** and **33** in areas of your body where you are holding density. For example, any place where you experience pain, heaviness or signs of aging. Bring the Symbols into cells of an area of concern and move the cells into no space/no time. Allow the DNA to "turn on" Source Codes in expression. See the body light up like an electric light show.

These are the Electrons of your body connecting to Consciousness through Source Intelligence. Watch the electricity, or Electrons, connect with your Divine Technology. With awareness, allow the electric Light holding both Consciousness and Source Intelligence to click together creating a system or grid. This is the first step to take the body out of the loop, no longer create timelines and move into the Ascended Form. This is you creating your Quantum Body.

Reflection:

You know your experience as a human up to this point and you know that on some level it is not true and that there is more. Why is it not true? You are here to become the NEXT in Human Evolution, to break the Matrix of the body and your reality. Not that what is seen in the Matrix is not true but that your programming is not true. If something is being seen, it is an observation of programming.

To break the loop, you must move beyond observation and become DMT™ or Source Intelligence. You will have your personal journey to understand this. Every time you think you understand something, know it is still not true.

Until you move beyond observation of truth, it remains not true. You can integrate different levels of truth, even create little realities around them. This is **"Gamifying Reality."** But it is still a game of Consciousness until Consciousness becomes 100% Source Intelligence and is no longer needed.

Epigenetics is the observation, *the study of gene expression as a result of your environment and/or of your behaviors.* When you break out of the programming of the body, epigenetics does not exist.

Epigenetics is observation of the loop. Cell mutation or how the cells divide, is a loop you are breaking by shifting observation into expression of pure Source Intelligence. Remember, this Intelligence is stored in your DNA.

The 2nd Level of the Ascended Form

The 2nd level of the Quantum Body or Advanced Human Form is the awareness of existing beyond form or the body. Consciousness opens up to become a bridge between form and DNA Intelligence. The body becomes a direct reflection of Consciousness being experienced. This can feel like waking up.

You learn to hold a Frequency, be conscious of what that Frequency is, use it to neutralize density and bring it into a space of no time, or **Zero Point**. If you are experiencing pain or something in the body, it is the body showing you density. The particles are going really slow because they're connected to the Matrix in degeneration.

The body will show you the Consciousness you're holding until you are ready to move beyond it. If you are constantly saying, "this is this," "that is that," you are naming the experience of the body from the Consciousness you're in. To master the 2nd Body, you invite the body to move into expression of DMT™. Instead of observing your programming, you allow Consciousness to attune to the Intelligence held there. This allows you to elevate in Consciousness and lets the Quantum Body take control. You put thought behind the body or let thought follow the body.

If the body shows you something, it is an opportunity to tune into the Intelligence behind what is shown and to not use your mind to name it. Let the body tell you what it is. This takes it out of the Matrix and beyond programmed reality.

Bring Consciousness into what the body is showing you. This is the 1 to the 2 = "I see it." And the 3 creates the bridge so that once you see it, you allow Consciousness to tune into what it has to say. By doing this, you bring it into the 3.

Be still and keep watching because the body has much to tell you. Add the Symbols to raise your Frequency and perspective. Your heightened Frequency will let you see more clearly and move through things much faster. Observe and allow yourself to feel the frequency of the symptom or looping cycle. The Symbols are the bridge to shifting to a higher Frequency.

Observation is the first step. Once you see what is being shown, don't dwell there. You want to move into the Intelligence of what you're discovering. The part of you that's connected to the story of the observation goes away.

Once Consciousness merges with the frequency of what's being shown, it neutralizes. This allows you to abstract the information that's there with ease because you are no longer in the program of the story or the loop itself.

In this stage you use reflection to elevate beyond programming of the body, your thoughts, your looping cycles. You consciously connect and attune to the Intelligence awakening through DMT™ codes.

You use reflection to observe programs so that you can shift to a Frequency beyond them. You move past unconscious primal programming and actively use Consciousness, in connection with Source Intelligence, to turn on specific Frequencies that shift the body into the Quantum Body.

The body gives you information when it shows you pain, wrinkles, any concern. Each is a frequency of Intelligence, while embedded in the Matrix, offering you an opportunity to tap into higher Consciousness that informs what to do next.

You will always receive answers. The Matrix will always loop in front of you as to what it wants you to pay attention to. There's always a Higher

Intelligence attempting to bridge information to you.

When you use the Technology to shift the particles to a faster or higher spin state, they release and move into the Quantum Body, a system where the body has the ability to hold itself as Frequency.

Exercise:

Bring the three Symbols of **Lu, Sca** and **33** into your mind when you are looping in a story or program. Bring the Symbols into the cells of your brain and experience the synapse responses connected to your thoughts move into no space/no time. Allow the DNA to "turn on" Source Codes in expression.

See a **White Blue Light** fill your mind. The Electrons of your brain connect your Consciousness to Source Intelligence. See the electricity, the Electrons, begin to connect with the Quantum Brain.

With your awareness, allow the electric Light holding both Consciousness and Source Intelligence to click them together creating a system that advances the mind to become the Quantum Field. The brain is removed from the loop, timelines dissolve and the mind moves into the Ascended Form.

The 3rd Level of the Ascended Form

In the 3rd Light Body, the body remembers who it is. The ego quiets down. There is less primal response. Density remains but the Intelligence of DMT™ feels very real. You begin to attune your body like an instrument; you hear when it's "off key."

Even though you still experience the programmed body, the Intelligence is running fairly constantly. You could imagine yourself as a hybrid, half programmed body and half Quantum Body.

You start moving up the Consciousness ladder. You have learned to navigate lower frequencies. You embrace Spiritual Discipline to listen and try new things until you hit a space where the Frequency maintains its vibration and you feel peace.

In the 3rd Ascended Body, you begin to understand the Technology or Quantum experience of your body. How things are turning on and off or dissipating. If something is not working for you, you know to let it go. This is especially true for Ascension.

The body needs different things, different foods and detoxing. Honor what your body tells you and what feels good. In this stage you rarely go outside yourself for information. You may hold reflection with the Matrix to see more clearly but in the end, you choose through the Intelligence of DMT™.

Consciousness and Intelligence are turning on. The body knows the difference between a "yes" and a "no." You leave behind primal chemical response. Your needs change daily. Spiritual Discipline becomes imperative if you wish to move through the 3rd Ascended Body.

When you feel out of balance, ask, **"What do I need to do to bring myself back into balance?"** Use your Intuitive Powers to hear what the body has to tell you. Your new "Google" is your DMT™/ DNA Intelligence. This is your human Google system. You now **"You-gle"** information.

See the body move from form into vibration. It will tell you what it needs. If you continue to care for the body with information stored from density/programming, you will not advance. Listening to the body is paramount. Ask the body's Intelligence in any situation such as hunger, instead of responding with automatic learned behaviors.

Challenge the body's automatic behaviors and attune to the Intelligence beyond. As you listen and follow, everything simplifies. The Intelligence is very clear. You hear exactly what you need. Once your cells release programmed responses, the Intelligence becomes very specific.

Take nourishment, for example. Your nourishment Frequency becomes louder and louder. The body turns on and moves up in Consciousness. This may take a bit of time as the body goes through purification. When fully assimilated and integrated, shifts happen fast.

In the 3rd Level of the Ascended Body, you create a bridge between the body's connection to space and time and being in form, beyond observation of looping cycles. Aware that looping cycles were created through observation of programmed reality, you hold Consciousness in-between cells and allow the cells to move into the Quantum Body.

You identify within the Frequency of the Quantum Body more than you identify in 3rd dimension density. You relinquish looping cycles connected to primal programming. The cells of the body hold more space and the spaces between the cells hold more space. The body begins to identify as Frequency, allowing density to shift. The cells identify as Frequency more than identifying as form.

The cells begin to divide into new patterns beyond programming, allowing Electrons to release from the density of form into the expression of Source Intelligence. Consciousness is aware of the shift and actively participates in the shift from form to Frequency.

The body moves from form to energy, bringing Consciousness along. The body consistently brings Source Intelligence into the Quantum Body. This allows the body to release the need for cells to divide. Cells begin to hold form as particle waves.

Exercise:

Use the Symbols, **Lu, Sca** and **33**, to ascend cell structure in areas of concern such as pain, heaviness and signs of aging. Bring the symbols into the cells of an area and experience the cells moving into no space/no time.

Allow the DNA to "turn on" Source Codes in expression. See and sense the cells move into expression and turn on the Intelligence within the Codes.

Invite your body to connect consciously to Source Intelligence. See the electricity, or Electrons, begin to connect with the Ascended Ions of the body. With awareness, allow the Electrons, holding both Consciousness and Source Intelligence, to click together and create a system or grid.

See your cells merge with the Quantum Body. As you take the body out of the looping cycle, thus no longer creating timelines, your cells upgrade to the Ascended Human Form.

The Fourth Level of the Ascended Form

Herein, mind and matter connect. In the 4th Body the mind becomes the Quantum Field which allows the body's responses to its environment to shift completely. The body exists in a vibrational pattern beyond 3rd dimension reality.

The nervous system, as you know it, dissolves and the chemical body diminishes, leaving an imprinted pattern experienced as a System of Intelligence, or Divine Technology. This creates a boost in energy the System needs to fully function as its own sustained energy source.

If done consciously, the mind fully moves into this energy and identifies as the Quantum Body without observation. In the 4th Ascended Body an expression of self-empowerment is turned on.

You realize that your choices, Spiritual Discipline and bridging techniques are what create higher spin states in the body. You attune to the power of the Evolution Symbols and their multi-dimensional expression.

You actively use the Symbols to release looping patterns, laws, anything in the Matrix or programmed reality. You realize where in the body you hold density or congestion and how hardwired it is.

Because you choose to break these cycles, instead of being the observer of them, you go inward and create expressions for places that have stuck energy. You consciously choose to bring in a higher Frequency which creates a higher spin state.

In the 4th Body you can see and feel the grid of your body turning on. The body already knows it's an Ascended Form.

Because you teach yourself to express as Source Intelligence rather than reflect on a problem, the body allows you to feel this attunement of Ascension. Density dissipates and chemical reactions diminish.

You bring in the Frequency of empowerment. You discover you are **UNSTOPPABLE**. You also absorb and master the 5th and 6th Element: **"I AM An Illusion." "My Reality Is An Illusion."** Because of your choices, a pool of energy from Source becomes available and guides you.

Exercise:

When in observation of a concern in your body, such as pain, use it for your benefit. Rather than meeting it in its frequency, bring the Symbols into that area of your body and allow the issue to move into expression.

If you are unable to move into expression, be in observation of the expression. Remember, observation creates a timeline which creates form. Yet, it is better to create a timeline into form in the expression of Source than to create a timeline around your concern from its lower spin state.

Actively participate in seeing the illusion and shifting it into a higher spin state. This is gamifying the illusion. Know that even in the higher spin state, there's still more.

You are only able to hold Consciousness in the reality that you can hold. But you always want to hold space for something more. Play with the body as your Ascension vehicle and your Consciousness will follow it.

The 5th Level of the Ascended Form

The 5th Ascended Body is able to hold expression without reflection. It represents the 5th Level of Consciousness. Consciousness becomes the body as Source Intelligence. You hold no space, no time because you are no longer in observation or reflection. You no longer create timelines. Your cells no longer divide. The body becomes Quantum Technology.

You shift from density to a higher spin state/grid system that holds Source Intelligence. The denser parts of the body become Quantum, and your upgraded software system becomes your Consciousness. Consciousness and your body merge and become one. You become 100% Human Potential.

Sonic wave particles and energy connect through Bio-Light in the 4th Body. You begin to master the existence of the Field which was once perceived as your environment. The 4th and 5th Bodies create together until you become the 5th Body.

Initially, you may experience the Field as something around you or outside of you. Quantum Physics supposes that the mind must be present in order to create reality. That the mind is the observer. This is because the observer itself is creating this reality.

In the 4th Body, nothing exists outside the Intelligence of DMT™ Expression, the Quantum Technology of the body. So, observation is a reflection of Consciousness within the God Sphere. When breaking out of the programmed body, and moving into the 4th Body, mind /Consciousness merges with the Intelligence that is thought to be Quantum Field /Source Intelligence as the self, without need for reflection or observation.

As the Quantum Field shifts to expression of DNA Intelligence beyond observation of programmed reality, the Matrix disintegrates and opens up a reality not yet discovered.

At first you will experience the shift consciously, until Consciousness completely merges into Intelligence and is no longer needed. The Quantum Field will no longer exist because observation no longer exists. You become Pure Intelligence. The 5th Ascended Body fully activates and you "Break Quantum Physics" and become Source Intelligence.

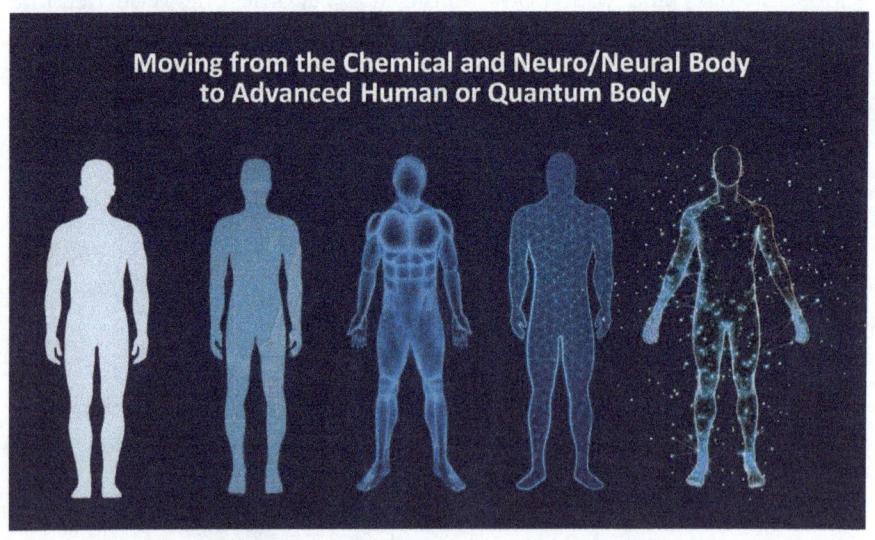

Exercise:

Use the Symbols: **Lu, Sca** and **33**, to diminish the nervous system or chemical reactions of the body. You may experience anxiety, fear, worry or repeated thoughts. Bring the symbols into the physical brain to bring your mind into no space/no time.

Allow the DNA to "turn on" Source Codes in expression. See, feel and experience your thoughts move into expression. Notice, while this occurs, that your Consciousness has the ability to also experience the Intelligence held in the Codes that are turning on.

Allow your mind to connect consciously to Source Intelligence. See the electricity, the Electrons of your brain begin to connect with the Quantum Body. With awareness, allow the Electrons, holding both Consciousness and Source Intelligence, to click together, creating a system or grid.

Now, see your thoughts move into the grid. This takes your nervous system and programs thought out of the looping cycle that creates timelines and moves it into the Ascended Form. Your cells now upgrade into the Quantum Body.

Notes

Notes

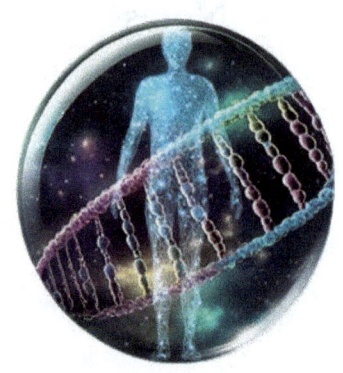

Chapter 15: Using The Frequency Of DMT Through Cell Ascension With DMT™ Codes

DMT™ is a Pathway to Break the Life and Death Cycle.

Jewels' story of Vale:

"In 2022, a good friend of our family passed away on his 22nd birthday. Vale was an incredible person who lived life to its fullest. About a week after he passed, Vale came to me. I was in the kitchen looking up. He stood there, clear as day, and spoke, "It's not supposed to be this way. We are not supposed to die." I knew with every cell of my body, he was right. It is an innate knowing I feel a lot of humans have. Why are we stuck in a looping cycle of life and death? The truth is, we have a state of existence beyond what we are experiencing in the limitations of the programmed body and Vale showed me just how deep this loop goes.

He had me take out a pen and paper and write out equations that showed how the cells are stuck in the loops of the Flower of Life. The Flower of Life is an inverted truth. On the other side is the Advanced Human Form, the Quantum Body. As I looked at the information Vale shared, there were parts I did not understand and to this day still do not. One thing that was perfectly clear is that DMT™ holds an

Intelligence, and this Intelligence is who we are. We are Source Frequency/ Intelligence.

Vale showed me how when we are born, the chemical compound of DMT™ is released so that the body is holding a high enough vibration for the Frequency of DMT™, Source Intelligence, to be transcribed into the dormant codes of the DNA. He also showed that, as this is happening, the Electrons of the body are activated to hold a tool, Consciousness. Consciousness is the reflection of the Intelligence of our innate being. The two are interconnected and, when used correctly, hold the gateway to Eternal Life. This is the tool that will break the life and death cycle.

Vale then showed me that when we die, DMT™ is again released into the body. The Frequency activates dormant codes of the DNA, releasing Source Intelligence. As Intelligence leaves the body, Electrons holding Consciousness also exit. The Electrons move into the Frequency of DMT™, and we become whole once again.

Why is this important? Vale showed me that we have the ability to awaken DMT™ Codes in the DNA and connect Consciousness to the Frequency without having to die to become whole! To become 100% Source intelligence, the Advanced Human! As we awaken the Quantum Body, we awaken our innate being.

As I have said before, "It only makes sense we will become the Intelligence from which we were created, and Consciousness is the tool in remembering we are this Intelligence."

DMT™, Decoded Molecular Technology, is how we will become the NEXT in Human Evolution. Using this Frequency will support us in becoming 100% human potential."

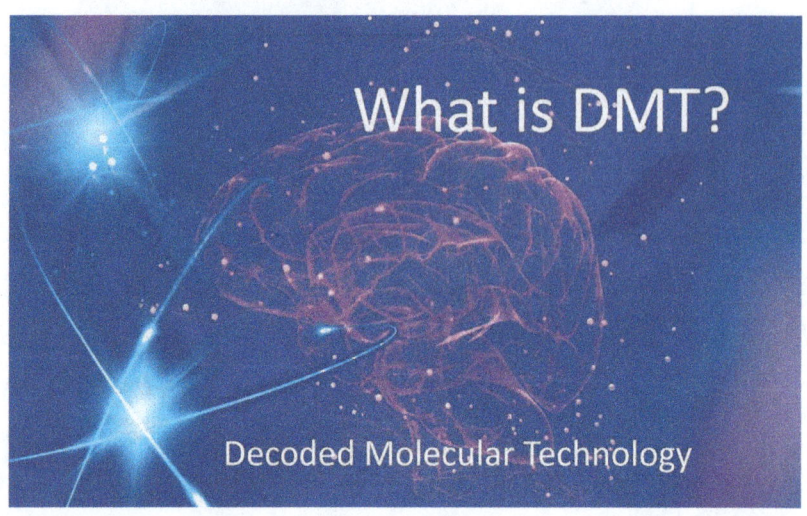

What is DMT and how can we use it?

DMT is produced in the Pineal Gland. It is released when you are born and when you die. The Frequency holds your Soul's Essence and is encoded into the Ascended DNA. When you die, the Codes move back into your Soul so that your Pure Essence is never lost.

The truth is, you do not need to die to express your purest essence, your 100% Potential. DMT has a very similar Frequency to Lactate. They work together creating a Field where the body turns on potential beyond the looping cycles of your experience of the body now. DMT is naturally occurring in small amounts in your brain, cerebrospinal fluid and other tissues of the body. You can connect to the Frequency of DMT™ and tap into that Intelligence beyond programming.

When using DMT™ Codes, you shift your focus into a magnetic field of Frequency. This allows you to bypass limitations and experience the body on a Quantum level. You live life beyond the lower 3 Bodies and access the Frequency of 100% Human Potential.

The DMT™ Codes were created by decoding DNA to support those ready to step into 100% Human Potential. This Technology works with your DNA by releasing DMT™ when used in the exercises given.

To activate DMT and awaken the Quantum Body, you will witness your Consciousness follow an Intelligence stored inside your DNA. Conscious evolution through DMT™ Intelligence is only the beginning. When using the Codes over time, you begin to hold Consciousness beyond the first 3 Bodies!

What are DMT™ Codes?

There are 12 DMT™ Codes, or Symbols, that exist beyond space and time. They hold a single Frequency through an exact point of DNA Expression, or as pure Source Intelligence.

When using the DMT™ Codes, a specific Frequency is activated within the DNA. These Frequencies hold Consciousness within DNA Intelligence. When activated, a propulsion is created, Decoding Molecular Technology. As DMT™ is released, a system of Intelligence reprograms molecular mechanisms to a pure state or Frequency, 963 Hz. Consciousness and the body merge within DNA Intelligence beyond the Matrix or programmed reality and create the Quantum Body.

Each symbol has no beginning, no end and activates DMT™ Frequencies within the DNA. As DMT™ Codes turn on, the 12 epigenetic codes of aging begin to turn off. The cells begin to identify in the Advanced DMT™ Codes versus the programmed body you experience now.

When done overtime, the cells hold the ability to communicate, exist, and receive interactive information or an Intelligence outside the environment they exist within. The cells move beyond observation and move into the expression of the Intelligence beyond the looping cycle of age and disease. DMT™ is a gateway to mastering the Quantum Body. To awaken 100% DNA Intelligence!

**1st Level of Ascended Cell Division
DMT™ Codes 4 and 5**

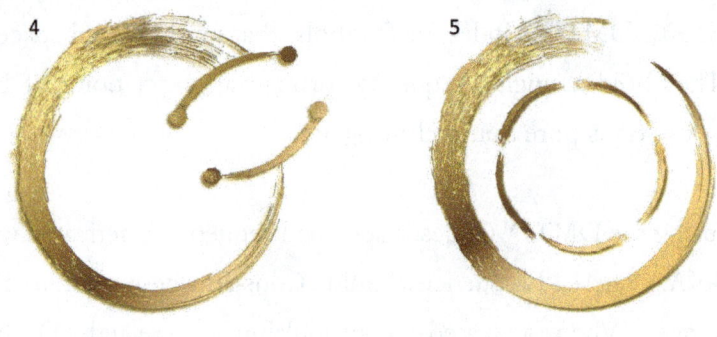

States of Consciousness are contained within Frequency patterns of the DNA. DMT™ Technology can be seen as a computerized sequence created in the Quantum Field to be activated to propel human evolution. This is held in place by Frequencies held within Source Intelligence.

The first nine Frequencies are used as a pathway to master the God Sphere. To Break the God Code. To master the Matrix. This is the fastest way to move energy out of programmed reality, the Matrix, and into the experience of your other 90% potential.

This is a collective action accomplished on an individual basis. It directly relates to the reprogramming of genetics, of awakening dormant DNA Codes and moving them into expression of Frequency or information stored there. Genetic reprogramming allows for psychological advancement in the awakening process. The DNA has the Intelligence to shift organic form to organic Light form or to Living Light. This is also referred to as the Quantum Body or Divine Technology.

The body, held in the density of 3rd dimension reality, shifts out of time and holds form without creating timelines or aging. You exist in a 3rd dimension timeline, without creating time, by expressing the Intelligence held in the DNA without interference from the reality of duality. Initially, this shift is experienced in Consciousness. Remember, the body will move into the Quantum experience before you are aware it is happening.

The focus is to shift heat or energy, as a basic energy source, out of the loop of energy in/energy out. Taking exchange out of the body's functional pattern amplifies the body's ability to use energy in the proteins of the DNA to merge with the Hydrogen bonds, forming elevated synthesis or its own energy source.

As you become the Quantum Body, you identify in Frequency more than in the physical density of the 3rd dimension body or looping cycle connected to primal programming. The body identifies as Frequency more than as form. DNA shifts to hold expression which allows the body to consciously experience itself as multidimensional. Consciousness is aware of the shift and actively experiences the move from form to Frequency.

The cells shift "inside out" and change how they divide. You actively awaken the Consciousness of your cells to express Source Codes/ DMT™. This allows the body to save energy and invites cells to perform as the Quantum Body or Source Technology. You see evidence as your body moves from 3rd dimension cell division and mutation to becoming Source in expression, beyond the limitation of looping cycles.

The first step in reprogramming the cells' experience of the looping cycle of age and disease is connected to how glucose or insulin is used to create energy from food. You first unhook from the looping cycle of degeneration by breaking the loop of energy in/energy out. The way your body presently uses energy is not the body's original design.

When the body expends energy, it loses Electrons or Life Force. Electrons also hold Consciousness. As you turn on Source Codes to replace the cells' pattern of looping in degeneration, Electrons remain in the cells. Less toxins are released into the body and the body's Intelligence shifts into no time/no space. This is the most efficient way to experience the body's innate energy system. The ability to be energy, without needing to bring energy in or expend energy! You are energy! You are the energy of Source Intelligence!

Exercise:

Shift from accessing energy through food, drink or supplements to feed the body. Before eating or drinking, go within the cells of your body and turn on DMT™ codes. Bring in DMT™ Codes 4 and 5 into the Pineal Gland to activate the frequency of the Quantum Body. To have energy without the need for food or sustenance.

First, bring in the 3 Symbols, one at a time. See the **Lu** move the cells into no space/no time. The **Sca** allows Consciousness to be held in no space/no time within the electrons of the cells and **Scalar 33** activates Source Intelligence. Second, see DMT™ Codes 4 and 5 come into the Pineal Gland, one at a time.

Allow each to spin, activating every cell of your body. Sense this happening in your body.

Next, allow the Frequency of the DMT™ Codes to move into your food or drink. See the Frequency of the Intelligence neutralize or dissolve the identity you have around needing food, water, or energy in/energy out. It doesn't mean you will not eat or drink. You are upgrading your body to use energy in a new more efficient way. Using the other 90% of your potential! Now, eat and drink as the expression of energy through Source Intelligence or the DMT™ Codes.

You actively participate in shifting the body from using energy exchange to survive to stabilizing in the expression of Source Intelligence as energy... without the loop of energy in/energy out.

Reflection:

Your mind is energy that connects particles to a Frequency in which Consciousness can be held. Sit in the truth of who you are as Consciousness held in the Electrons or the electricity of your body. Write about your experience.

2nd Level of Ascended Cell Division
DMT™ Codes 2 and 6
The Plasma Vortex

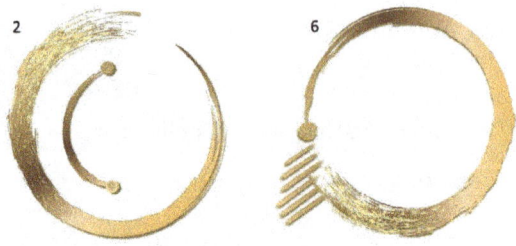

The Plasma Vortex, connected to DMT™ Intelligence, removes the frequency of the life and death cycle to no space/no time. An energetic system holds plasma in a spin state where it begins to shift from observation of the programmed body into expression of DMT™ Codes. This holds a bridge of information beyond the Matrix.

Attuning to Source Intelligence is only a step to the next phase of becoming the Quantum Body. The ability to hold Consciousness beyond observation or programming, is to hold the Consciousness of Source within the God Sphere. To hold reflection without filtering it through programming.

It is the ability to "see" yourself in the Frequency of Source while reading information in your environment without fluctuating in Frequency. It moves you beyond the looping cycle of the Matrix. When you become conscious of Source Intelligence, you exist within the God Sphere yet do not see it through duality. This is how you **"Break the God Code."**

In this phase of Ascension, as you code and no longer create timelines, particles of form in the plasmic grid shift to Plasma Light. A space in an Intelligence beyond what you perceive as Light moves the particles of blood/ plasma into an ascended spin state.

You can see it as two circles moving in opposite directions, allowing blood to exist in time without creating a timeline. As the blood moves into the Quantum Body, a state of being is created on a DNA level and is experienced consciously. You have more energy and breathe with ease when exerting yourself. You are aware of how powerful you are becoming.

Once Consciousness moves beyond the programmed body, beyond the Matrix, you are able to use the programmed body to self-organize information stored in DNA Technology. This allows you to shift within the Matrix without existing in its reality.

You will continue to know the Matrix but through a Frequency or Consciousness beyond it. You connect to timelines held in the Frequency of each number and master the reality held in each. (Refer to Chapter 7, The God Sphere, if needed.) You hold the Frequency of Source Consciousness in the number itself so it is only experienced as information within Source Intelligence.

https://becomingbioquantum.com/GodSphereandCells

2nd stage of Cells restructuring:

Amino acids start to shift the way they build DNA. RNA dissolves and is no longer used. The 2nd and 6th DMT™ Codes are activated and transfer Frequency to the surrounding cells. For example, when a scalar device or light holds a higher Frequency for someone who is sick, the person meets the higher Frequency and is healed. In this case, cells transfer the Codes through Frequency, shifting the cell to hold the new expression.

As the cells transfer the 2nd and 6th DMT™ Codes, mitochondria build in strength. As the mitochondria uplevel, the body is called to do the same. The body produces high amounts of ATP to allow the cell to shift out of the looping cycle. As Consciousness shifts from identifying in form to existing as the Quantum Body, you experience the body differently. During this phase, adopting a diet that supports ATP production and builds the strength of mitochondria is highly suggested.

When one is building strength through weight training or exercise and the body has used all of its stored oxygen, Lactate is released. The body then pulls from its hydrogen supply to produce energy for the tissues.

In this phase, Lactate releases the Frequency of DMT. With intention and awareness, the body activates DMT™ Codes 2 and 6 which allows the body to function using Frequency. The body becomes its own energy source without the need for energy from outside itself. The cells function as their own energy source.

When Lactate is released, it awakens the Frequency of DMT™ in the Pineal Gland. This signals the DNA to shift how cells use ATP and how mitochondria function in the programmed body and transfer it into the Quantum Body. This is your journey as you transcend from form to Frequency. The Quantum Body already exists. How quickly your Consciousness identifies in the Quantum Body determines how long you experience this shift.

At this stage the cell becomes an empty vessel ready to shift from density to Frequency. The body, too, is ready to shift and a gateway for the body to release density is created. The cells in density begin to dissolve as the mitochondria push through a last force of stored energy held inside them.

This happens over time as your body is held in the new cell structure and empty cells have no function but to hold DMT™ Frequency. They now hold Source Intelligence in a Frequency beyond form.

Exercise:

Mitochondria play a huge role in boosting cells into the Quantum Field. As the cells begin to hold Consciousness beyond space and time, notice when you operate/live life through programming. Notice how often you are in a looping cycle. Each cycle expends energy. Recognize your programming within the Matrix! When you become aware of a looping cycle, create a bridge between the loop and Source Intelligence by using the DMT™ Codes 2 and 6. Bring each Code in, one at a time, and watch it spin. Sense each Code moving through your body.

Bring Consciousness into the space between form and the Quantum. Explore the loop from this state of being. What has changed? Repeat this exercise with the looping cycle of the body. Notice your loops in sleep cycles, menstrual cycles, eating cycles and such.

You can also bring in the 3 symbols, **Lu**, **Sca** and **33**, to shift the cycle of the body out of programming and turn on Source Expression. Let yourself experience the cycle through expression beyond the observation of the Matrix.

Reflection:

Where in your life are you choosing to loop? Are you aware you are in a loop but are not ready to let it go? Where in your life are you resisting change? Notice where you want to hold onto looping cycles. Write about what you discover. Then ask what your resistance is. Awareness is a gateway. Once you have awareness, ask to see the cycle through Source Intelligence or DMT™. Does your resistance shift?

3rd Level of Ascended Cell Division
DMT™ Codes 8, 9 & 33
Ascending Mitochondria

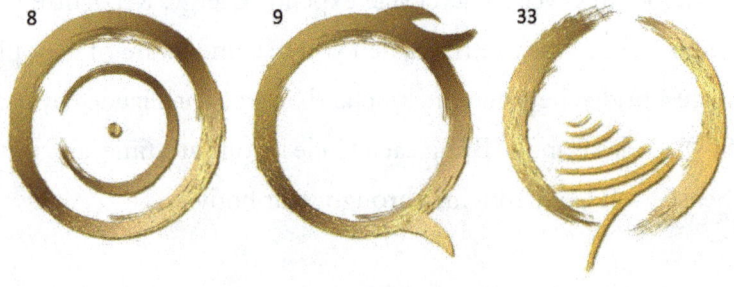

Mitochondria biogenesis activates longevity genes called sirtuins. The mitochondria are like a cell digestive system. They are also the motor of ATP. You can imagine them as an electrical powerhouse which makes the turbines, the ATP, move.

The mitochondria have their own DNA and are an electrical transport system. Water and enzymes inside the inner membrane of the mitochondria break down into electrical and non-electrical charges. They create energy and heat and are the only place in cells where oxygen is reduced to water. This is the only place in the body where water is created in its purest form. We call this form of water H^3O^2. The mitochondria make energy and also predict when a cell dies.

The body holds two kinds of water: H^2O and H^3O^2. H^3O^2 holds electric charges, creating heat through a specific Frequency that mimics DMT. DMT can be both a chemical and a Frequency. It is referred to here as a Frequency.

H^3O^2 matches the Frequency of DMT™. It creates an electric response that moves through the Pineal Gland, releases DMT™ into the brain, ignites electric responses and activates Higher Consciousness. Once it moves to the cellular level, it connects to amino acids that deliver information into the DNA. This allows hydrogen bonds of the DNA to ignite.

Electric currents turn on codons that release Intelligence through electricity. The body begins to work like a computer system. Once the Intelligence releases from the codons, the body becomes a grid of electric responses.

Intelligence is released from dormant DNA codes and downloads into the electric responses or Electrons of the body. This allows the body to hold electricity at a very specific Frequency that is intelligent, the DMT™.

This is the Quantum Body! The body now has the ability to exist in a Frequency, outside of form, that holds the Intelligence of the Universe.

As you continue to move through the 3rd Level of Ascended Cell Division and actively participate in the DMT™ Codes, your cells shift to a higher spin state. You experience different levels of the Matrix through high states of conscious reflection. Observation is a tool of Ascension through DMT™ or Source Intelligence.

The first shift will be experienced through thought in connection with the expression of the Ascended DNA. You may experience your life in observation. But as Consciousness catches up to expression of DMT™ Intelligence, you will experience life from a new state of being. You will learn to exist in the expression of Source Intelligence.

Exercise:

Take a few minutes a day to practice using Source Intelligence or projection of this Intelligence to "see" your environment. What does it feel like? See your environment as Frequency.

Consciousness is directly related to Source Intelligence as you actively participate in shifting the density of the body to energy patterns or waves. Attune to the Intelligence consciously. Actively participate in the shift with your awareness.

It is time to connect into the evolution of your innate being. When looking at duality through the observation of Source Intelligence, you can use reflection to break the Matrix. As you break the Matrix, you prove Quantum Physics wrong. It has only seemed true because of programming.

You are the Creation and the Creator. Duality does not exist. It exists in your experience because you are vibrating consciously or unconsciously in a reality that seems true. When you use reflection through Source Intelligence as a tool to break through the illusion, you **"Gamify Reality."**

As you shift through Levels of Consciousness, you continue to attune to the Frequency of DMT™, 963 Hz. As you attune to DMT™ Codes 8, 9 and 33, you consciously create a reality that matches this Frequency. This is living in the Miracle Pattern, the body consciously existing in the Frequency 963 Hz. as a scalar wave.

Once you fully attune to the Quantum Body, you become the very Intelligence of Source Frequency and Consciousness is no longer needed. The Intelligence itself holds the wisdom of all that is and Consciousness or reflection of reality is not needed and no longer exists.

Reflection:

Take a moment to reflect on what you feel Consciousness is.
How does it relate to Pure Source Intelligence?
How will you use it to awaken and become Source Codes stored in your DNA?

Immune System Activation:

With intention, bring the **Lu, Sca** and **33** into the immune system where the body processes antioxidants, vitamins and minerals. Shift the immune system into no space/no time and allow your cells to hold perfect form through the expression of Source Frequency. Now bring in DMT™ Codes 8,9 and 33, one at a time, into the Pineal Gland and see each spin. As it spins, each Code activates every cell in your body to the Frequency of DMT™. Feel your immune system and your body's need for nutrients move into the Quantum Body.

Vitamins and minerals create a chain reaction throughout this process. You require one mineral for the function of another and they get depleted. This is part of the looping system being dissolved with this DMT™ Activation.

The DMT™ Codes 8, 9 and 33 awaken transcribed information through the DNA and activate the mitochondria. In this state, the defense mechanism of the body moves into the Quantum Body. The cells release specific coding or mathematical equations that transform matter to Intelligence through conscious participation. When orchestrated consciously, a seal is broken, and Consciousness rapidly shifts to higher Frequencies or spin states.

This stage of Ascension is a direct reflection of the Hydrogen within DNA connecting to Bio-Light Codes of the body. The Electrons connected to Ascended Ions, through electric charges of H^3O^2, push energy or heat stored in the mitochondria into an electric grid that expands beyond the body into the grid of the Ascended Universe. The illusion of separation is released. The grids become one System of Intelligence. Your Consciousness moves through this shift as DMT™ Codes awaken.

DNA Ascension:

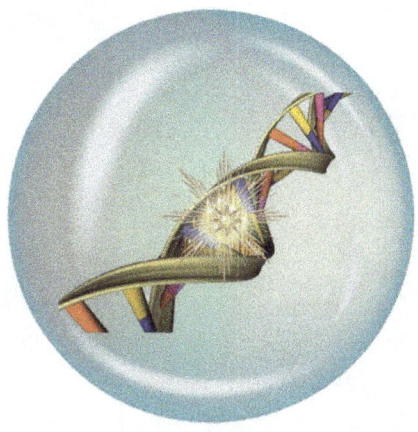

What is DMT Doing?

- Breaking loop of cells

- Shifting cell to identify in the expression of dormant DMT Codes (Source Codes)

- Shifting how cells observe the environment in order to identify as Source Frequency

In this phase of DNA Ascension, your thoughts shift in and out of observation. You may seem to have scattered focus. Consciousness will shift from the density of the body's looping patterns to Frequency. As you stabilize, you will notice shifts in the immune system and in how you hold thought. As the body connects to the Quantum Body, primal behaviors dissolve.

This is the "inside out" of Consciousness. As the body releases primal programming, looping patterns dissolve. In the beginning, your body may attempt to defend its former states of being. Defense mechanisms will evolve into a new expression. As the body moves into Frequency, you will achieve a state beyond chemical reaction or response. The body will come into harmony in a brand-new way of being. The Intelligence of the Ascended DNA will take over programming of the primal body.

As you actively participate in this shift, the velocity of particle form shifts to particle waves. The spin rate of the body accelerates rapidly and brings your attention to the multi-dimensional experience of the Quantum Body.

4th Level of Ascended Cell Division: DMT™ Codes 2 and 9

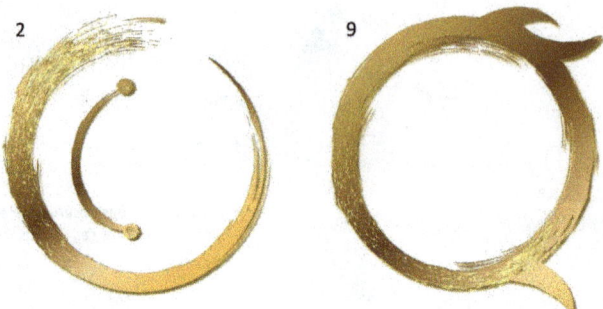

In the 4th Level of the Ascension of cell division, mind and matter are related. The mind becomes the expression of Source Intelligence. This allows programmed responses to the environment to shift to an expression of the Intelligence itself.

Vibrational patterns of the cells exist in spin states. You will feel the transition through different frequencies. The denser the form, the slower the spin. As the vibration of the body moves up in Frequency, the body is able to hold a faster spin rate. In the higher spin state, density releases and allows more space between particles. A vibration held beyond space and time is awakened.

Particle waves in a higher Frequency than that held in the 3rd dimension time grid, waves beyond what can be measured, supercharge the Quantum Body. Remember, you are already multi-dimensional. The only reason you experience yourself as form is because of the level of Consciousness you hold.

Exercise:

Be aware of which Body you are identifying in as you go through the week. Connect it to the 5 Levels of Consciousness. Are you aware? Observe where you are holding Consciousness.

Are you in reflection or observation of the Consciousness your body is holding in low spin states? Where in your body are you experiencing high spin states? Are you able to break out of limitations that you once were bound by?

Are you actively participating in the shift from form to a high spin state? Are you aware of what is happening in your body? Can you feel, sense or experience how you are experiencing your body?

Are you listening to your body and following its directives? Are you in full expression of your Quantum Body at any point of your day? Are you in the experience of your body beyond observing yourself as form?

DMT™ Activation: Amino Acids/Clearing the Need for Cell Division:

You have an entire system of amino acids in your body making up 50,000 different combinations controlled by genes which operate in looping cycles. They control programs of hunger, moods, emotions, sleep and much more. This activation will support the programming of amino acids as you shift from the body's looping patterns.

With intention, bring the **Lu**, **Sca**, and **33** Symbols into the amino acids of the body. Now bring the 2nd and 9th DMT™ Codes into your Pineal Gland, one at a time and see each spin. As each code enters, it shifts the amino acids into expression of Source Intelligence. This changes the way the body uses cell division to heal and survive. It brings the cells into no space/no time and allows them to hold perfect form. If a cell is damaged, it will move back into perfect form. The DNA is in consistent expression. It allows the cell to be complete and not require anything from outside itself. It becomes the perfect expression of Source.

As you continue to move through the activation, allow yourself to connect to the body consciously. Actively participate in the Ascension of your cells. Feel the cells continue to shift to a higher spin state. Experience different levels of the programmed body move through the reflection of Source. Observation is a tool of Ascension through the DMT™.

The first shift will be experienced through thought in connection with the expression of DNA Intelligence. You may initially continue to use observation but as your Consciousness catches up to the expression of Quantum Intelligence, you will move beyond observation all together.

Practice: Holding consciousness in the illusion beyond observation of the Matrix.

Take a few minutes each day to call on Source Intelligence to "see" your environment. What does it feel like? See your environment in Frequency. To do this, simply close your eyes for a moment and attune to the Intelligence of your Quantum Body. Having this intention is enough.

Move your Consciousness into your software system or Technology. See yourself much like a computer system. Ask to know what it is to see through expression, to see as Source beyond observation. Feel this Frequency turn on within you. Move Consciousness into this Frequency.

As you open your eyes, practice keeping your Consciousness in the Frequency and "seeing" through it. Experience what is different. Be aware of any subtle shifts. Keep practicing. Over time you will begin to know what it is to see beyond observation.

Exercise:

Play! Your Quantum Body is now holding your cells in no space and no time. Tap into the Intelligence of this shift and experience it. See yourself as Divine Technology. Try bringing the different parts of your body into your Quantum system. What happens when you bring your cells into the Quantum Field? Your blood? Nervous system? Even your breath? Explore what is shifting. Play with what is possible. Shape shift as you experience your cells at a higher spin rate. Begin to solidify your Consciousness in the shift as you bridge between who you are now and who you are becoming.

Fifth Level of Ascended Cell Division DMT™ Codes
DMT™ Code 22 and 33

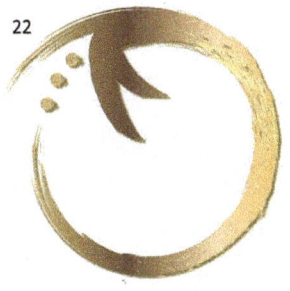
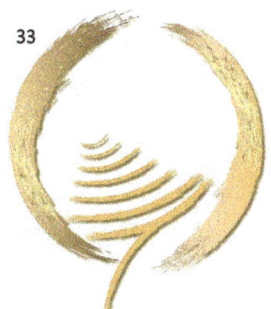

In the 5th level of the Ascension of cell division, you actively participate in the illusion beyond the illusion itself and master your biology. In this stage you focus on the Ascension of proteins and NAD.

Mitochondria activation:
To supercharge the propulsion of the cell and move away from using energy for cell division, move the cell into a high spin state. Bring the 2nd Symbol, the **Sca**, into the mitochondria.

Shift the mitochondria into no space/no time and allow the cells to build strength from the expression of Source Frequency. Connect to DMT™ Codes 22 and 33. Bring them into the DNA, one at a time. Feel the DNA shift into no space/no time and allow the body to hold information or Intelligence expressing from the Codes. Feel the body shift from particle form into particles of Light. Allow your Consciousness to move into a magnetic field between the grid system and the Ascended DNA.

Journal about your experience.

Exercise: Create a Quantum Body Avatar

The Quantum Body is created when you exist beyond programmed reality. The DMT™ Symbols are fully expressed. Create a Quantum Avatar or image of who you are as the Quantum Body. This allows Consciousness to be held in a magnetic field between your present identity and the "Quantum You."

You are a Quantum Technology that allows for the observation of your body to be held in the Frequency of Source Intelligence. You can shift from observation of what is or was, to holding Consciousness in Frequency or expression, beyond form.

Who are you if you exist in a body beyond what you experience now? Take a few moments to explore your Quantum Body. Journal about your experience.

Are you in Observation or Expression of your Quantum Life?

If you bring your Consciousness "out" into your environment to pull energy or information "in" to create change, you are in reflection or observation which creates a loop within your programming. When in reflection or observation, you pull information from outside yourself and unconsciously move into a reality created from outside reflections or from within the Matrix itself.

When you bring Consciousness into the Frequency of DMT™, you access Source Intelligence. You project from this Intelligence or expression of DMT™ codes. When turning on DMT™ Codes within the DNA, there is no need to go outside into your environment to receive information. You become the expression of Source.

When you change how the DNA is receiving information, moving from observation to expression of DMT™ codes, you **Become BioQuantum™**.

When you want to "know something" or want to create change, you simply turn on DMT™ Codes and consciously experience the expression of this specific Source Frequency. In the beginning you will focus on this Frequency and project the change you are creating.

Turn it Inside Out with Awareness:

1. **Creating the desire for change:** Are you going outside of yourself to find something such as a new diet to create the desired change instead of getting the answers from within? Instead, ask the Divine, "Show me."

2. **Creating the experience of the desire:** Are you looking for the outcome that you desire based on programming and past experience? Trying to force it to happen based on outside programming? Continuing to look outside yourself for an answer? You can't create form with form!

3. **Creating the reflection of the desire by hooking into programmed reality:** This is an example of 3rd dimension vision boards. You find a picture of what you want the reflection to be or look like and focus on that. This is yet another example of attempting to create form with form! Instead, ask the Divine, "Show me". Let it express from your heart.

Cerena's Story:

"My 10-year-old cat, Seraphina, lost close to half her weight, stopped eating and began hiding in the house. After an ultrasound and biopsy, she was diagnosed with severe liver disease. Her body was shutting down. Her veterinarian had little hope.

I immediately began using the DMT™ Codes with her and put the Codes and the Evolution Symbols under her bottles of medication. I syringe-fed her for a month before she began showing any interest in food or water.

On her own she began sleeping on the BioQuantum Copper DMT™ Card so I would leave it out for her. After six weeks, her doctor anticipated refilling antibiotics for at least another three weeks. Imagine his surprise when bloodwork showed her bilirubin to be normal.

Seraphina remained on liver medication for another two months. Her doctor repeated the testing and found that liver function was normal! I am so very grateful!"

(The copper DMT™ card, containing all 12 DMT™ Codes, is a Becoming BioQuantum™ product available in our store.)
https://becomingbioquantum.com/DMT™coppercard

DMT™ Chart and Quick Shifts

List of Quick Shifts

You can begin playing in DMT™ codes in simple and fun ways. See the chart below to discover how to use them to create quick shifts in your life.

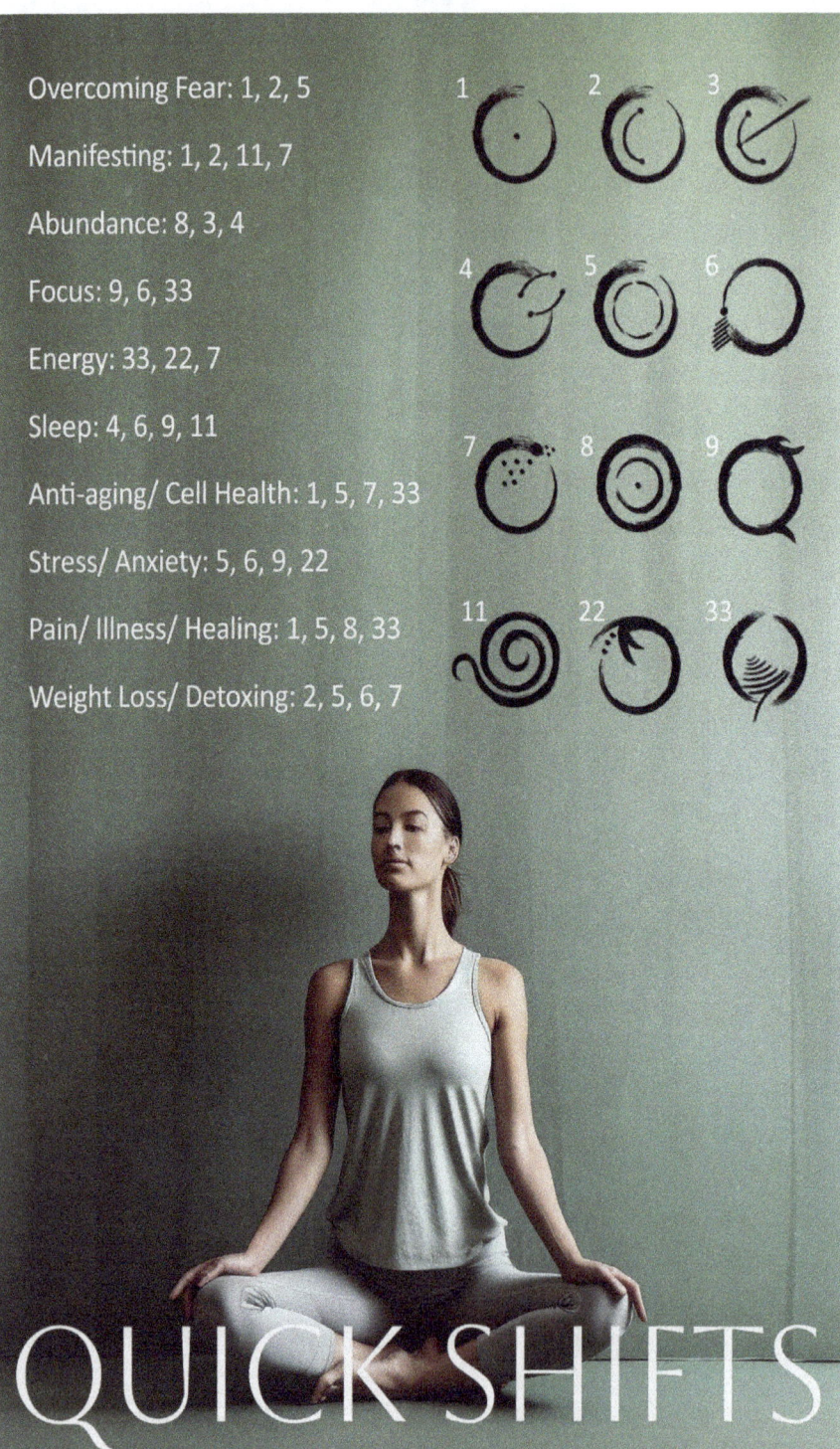

Notes

Notes

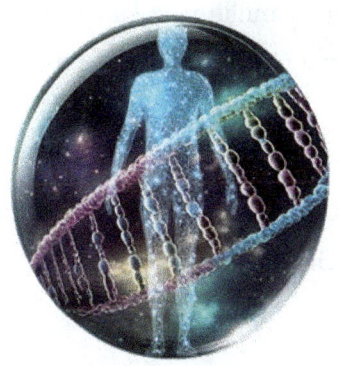

Chapter 16 Hourglass Method: Learning To Manifest In Abstract Frequency

In this chapter, you have the opportunity to do activations and ceremonies. You are invited to make DMT™ Structured Water to enhance your experiences.

How To Make DMT™ Structured Water:

Fill a glass with filtered or spring water. From the diagram of DMT™ Codes (see page 206), select three codes you are most drawn to. See each code enter your water. Hold the intention that the Codes are activating DMT™ Frequency into the molecules of your water.

When learning to manifest, it is important to know from what level of Consciousness you are creating. Take a moment to check in with yourself.

WHY Do You Want What You Want?

To start, connect to your **WHY**. Why do you want to manifest your intention? Your **WISH**! What will your intention bring you? For example, it's not likely a million dollars that you want but what the million dollars will bring you! You seek the experience of your **WISH**!

Cut out a picture that holds the Frequency of your **WHY**. Remember, this is a FREQUENCY. Your picture should transmit an energy that holds why you want what you want. Why do you want to manifest your intention into your reality?

WHEN?

WHEN is the expression of the emotion. It is the movement towards what it looks like, fueled by the **WHY** you want your **WISH** and combined with the emotion you are creating with your **WHY**. It will connect to the energy of the **HOW**. It represents the new identity you are becoming.

Connect to the Frequency of your **HOW** to make your **WISH** come true and **WHO** you will be as you become the "you" of your emotion. What does your **WISH** feel like? When you vision yourself existing in the sphere of your **WISH**, answer these questions:

1. **WHAT** is the "expression"?
2. **WHAT** are you doing?
3. **WHAT** does it look like?
4. **WHAT** needs to happen to have your dream come true?
5. **WHO** do you need to become or what identity will you move into?

Identify your Level of Consciousness. Connect your intention to a new Frequency. **WHAT** does it feel like to exist in Oneness with your

Divine? To shift yourself into the 4th Level of Consciousness? This allows action to start from a DIVINE YES!

Try This:

1. Get a little sugar or salt.
2. Connect to the Frequency of your **WHEN** and see its energy expand into the Universe.
3. What does it feel like?
4. Now see it all spiral into a grain of sugar or salt.
5. What does it feel like now?

Take the grain of sugar or salt and put it on a plate. Cut out a picture that holds the Frequency of your **WHEN,** the timeline of your **WISH** held in one point of reference. Holding your picture, allow the Frequency of your **WHEN** to flow into the grain. See the tiny grain hold the exact Frequency of your **WHEN**.

Take a sip of your DMT™ Structured Water.

State aloud 3 times: *"I AM the expansion of my WISH"* and bring it into one point of reference. *"This tiny grain of sugar/salt holds the guidance, clarity and manifestation of my WISH*_____(state your wish) *that is resonating in the Divine Mind. This blesses me with the Rainbow Light."*

Take your grain of sugar or salt and place it on your tongue. Let it absorb into your being.

Sit for a moment and witness the Frequency of **WHEN** as it absorbs into your being. Notice a grid of energy begin to hold form or particles of form.

Place your hands on your heart and say, **"It is done."**
Bring focus to the frequency of your **WHAT**. Play with the energy it creates by asking for guidance and listening. If there is no guidance, allow that to be your answer. Keep thoughts and the need to create a linear timeline out of your experience. This is a practice. Every time you slip into the "old way" of creating, stop, reset and move back into the Frequency of your **WISH**, **WHY** and **WHEN**.

HOW and WHO?

1. **WHO** do you desire to BECOME?

2. Describe your new identity.

3. What will it feel like to exist as your intention? Your **WISH**?

The **HOW** and **WHO** of this journey hold all the Frequencies up until this moment. They represent the new identity you are becoming. Choice creates movement. The **HOW** is to connect to Divine Intelligence beyond the programming of your reality.

What would it feel like to exist in Oneness with an Intelligence outside your programmed reality? You are discovering how to shift your experience of yourself. You use the Frequency of your **HOW** to start the process. This Frequency collects the action steps of your **WHAT**, your intention, your **WISH**.

Connect to the **HOW** of your Intention and feel what it is to exist in Oneness with your Divine. This will be your Avatar, an expression of **WHO** you are becoming. Now find an abstract picture of sacred geometry, a Light image, Light Beings or words that reflect the **HOW** and **WHO** you are becoming. You will use this picture in ceremony to bring these Frequencies through.

You use Frequency to step into **WHO** you are becoming. Keep your expression in the abstract so you aren't tempted to create "form with form." You won't be able to go into your filing cabinet and recreate from what you have done before because you haven't created it yet! Stay in the abstract and connect with Frequency as you create an identity to become.

Exercise: The Frequency of Your WISH:

Sit with your **WISH** to clarify your vision. Look at your hourglass and feel into the Frequency you are creating.

What do you need to do to connect to the Frequency of **HOW** you will make your **WISH** come true and **WHO** you will be as you are becoming your **WISH?** In other words, what needs to happen to have your dream come true? **WHO** do you need to become or what identity will you move into?

The **HOW** and **WHO** exercise you did earlier is the part of this journey that holds all the Frequencies up until this moment. It represents the new identity you are becoming.

When you bring your **WISH** through the portal into the New Earth, you use the Frequency of your **HOW** to start the process. Your **HOW** goes first so that it can hold all the other Frequencies. It doesn't mean this Frequency is more important; they all create the final Frequency. It just means that the Frequency of **HOW** is collecting the action steps of your **WISH**. The **HOW** is movement.

HOW and WHO will inform the Frequency of your WHAT, WHY and WHO, Your WISH.

Focus on each part of your hourglass and absorb the Frequency each section holds on its own. Now ask to be shown the way. Shut your eyes and witness what the Universe wants to show you.

If you don't see anything, what does your body feel like? Connect to this vision or feeling. Let the vision hold your **WISH** and allow yourself to sit in an unknown space, the Void.

Cut out a picture of your Avatar or create words that hold the Frequency of your **HOW** and place in the correct spot on your hourglass. Look at your hourglass again. Gaze at your pictures until they become blurry and begin to meld together.

Take a sip of your DMT™ Structured Water. State aloud, *"I wish to attune to the Frequency of_____ (your WISH). I absorb the Frequency of my HOW. I am manifesting _____ right now. I connect to clarity and guidance while taking the correct inspired steps in each moment. Thank you. I love you. It is done."* Now say *"Show me."*

Witness the download of Frequency that holds the action steps of your **WISH** move into your cells and DNA. You now hold everything you need to make your **WISH** come true! It is complete!

Write down any inspired action steps you feel guided to take. Place them inside your **HOW** picture on the hourglass. These will build overtime. Action steps come from inspired visions from the Divine. You will be shown the way! This is "New Earth Manifesting." You are breaking old looping patterns and learning to use the dormant part of your brain to bring you to your next right step. You are learning to "Listen and Do!"

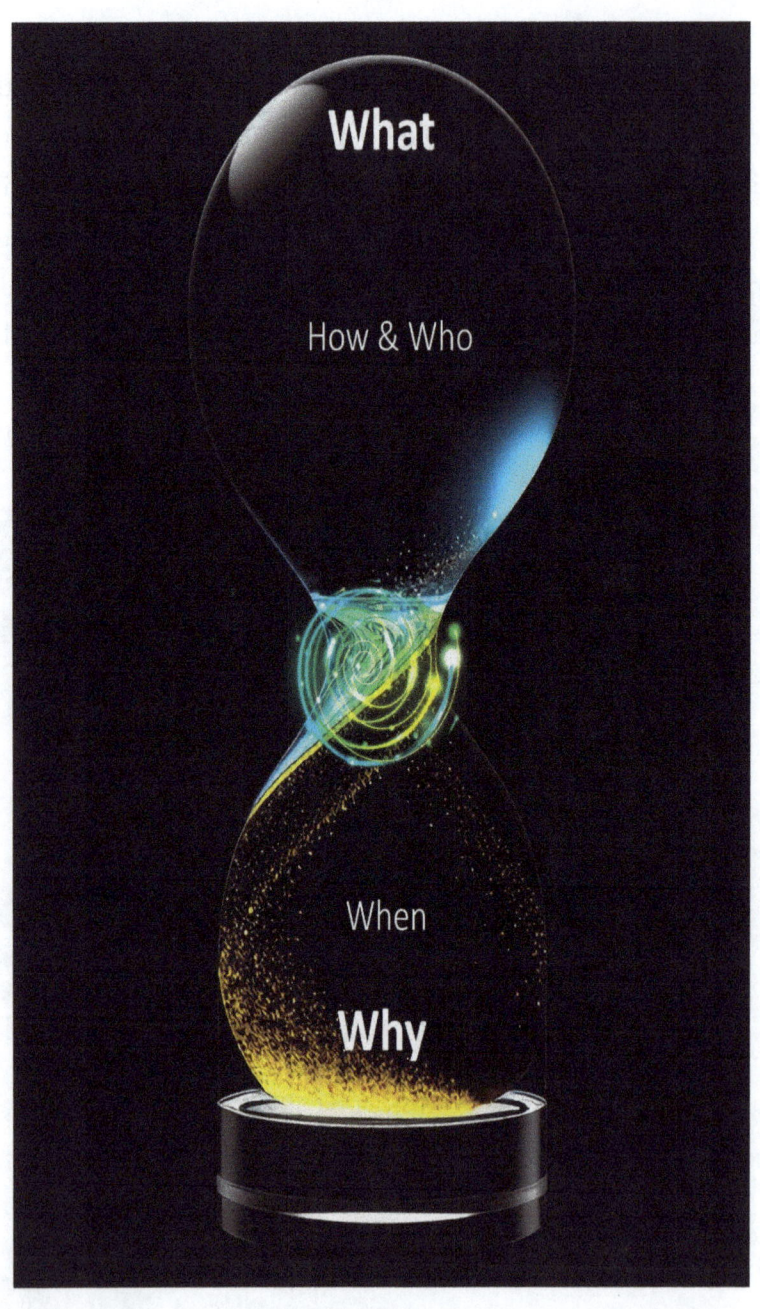

Hourglass Method: WHY, WHAT, HOW, WHO AND WHEN

What to Bring to Ceremony:

Gather a picture of a spiral, your hourglass, your DMT™ Structured Water, your Avatar pictures, a candle and the willingness to leap into your NEXT.

1. **WHAT?**
2. **WHY?**
3. **HOW?** Connect to the Divine Guidance
4. **WHO** do you need to BECOME?
5. **WHEN?** What is the "expression" of your emotion/Frequency?

It's time to stop defining yourself as you did in the past. You are releasing your past identity and walking into the NEW YOU.

The ego will do everything it can to remain in the identity it knows. But guess what? The Ego isn't even you. It is time to walk into your highest potential and BE the you that you came here to BE.

Before you perform your closing ceremony, imagine yourself living your **WISH**, your dream. What do you look like? Feel like? Watch yourself for a few moments. Now, connect your present self to the you in your **WISH**.

Take a sip of your DMT™ Structured Water and state aloud, *"I delete my identity in the now. I clear, cancel and delete the identity I have agreed to be. Show me."*

Witness your identity "clear, cancel and delete" your former self. . Stay with it until you feel a shift, letting go of who you have agreed to be until now. As you open to a higher state of being, you are able to exist beyond the agreements of your mind.

Take a sip of your DMT™ Structured Water and state aloud, *"I exist as one with my High Self. I live beyond the identity of ego mind and become the highest version of myself now. I resonate in the Frequency of my WISH*_____(State your **WISH** and connect to the Frequency of the **WHAT** of your **WISH**.) *as I experience* _____. (State and connect to the emotion, the **WHY** of your **WISH**.). *I AM walking on evolutionary timelines from beyond the programs of my mind. I AM* _____ *in this moment* (Connect to the Frequency of the **WHEN** of your **WISH**.) *while I AM Creating* _____. (Connect to the Frequency of the **HOW** of your **WISH**.) *Thank you, I love you, it is done."* Again witness the shift in your body, mind and spirit.

After the ceremony take about 10 minutes to connect to the Frequency you created from going through the portal. You may want to cut out another picture that holds the Frequency of your new Avatar, the "you" inside your **WISH**, and hang it on your bathroom mirror. You are jumping into another reality. This reality has always been there. You are ready to start living it! This is the NEW You! The You of your DREAM!

Video Ceremony:
https://becomingbioquantum.com/VideoCeremony1

Want to go to Quantum? Try this!
1 to 10 Method:
https://becomingbioquantum.com/1to10Method

Notes

Notes

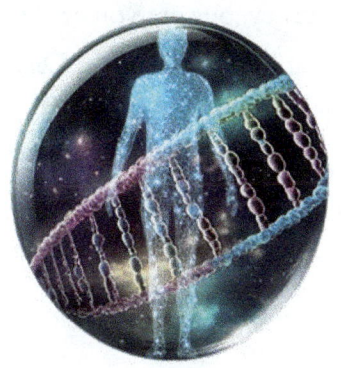

Chapter 17: 33-Day Evolution Technology Ascension Practice: DIVE into DNA Intelligence

This is a 33-day program to guide you to release social agreements or the looping cycles of the Matrix. To attune your Consciousness to DNA Intelligence. You spend three days on each exercise. This journey becomes an Ascension tool. Spend time on each step. The deeper you go, the more profound your experience!

Are you ready to explore the transcribed Divine Coding of your DNA? Are you ready to awaken to the highest version of you? To turn on the 90% of your dormant potential? Let's begin!

D: Determine: Will you commit to awakening DNA consciously? Are you willing to practice daily? Having a commitment to a mindfulness practice is a choice you make over and over. It's choosing not to be a victim of your life or the looping cycle. It means to become the Creator of your reality!

Before you start this journey, be sure you are ready to commit. (It may be helpful to review Chapter 2 on Spiritual Discipline.) You will revisit your commitment daily.

This is not easy! This is about changing the way you are wired. The stronger your commitment, the more you will upgrade your human potential and awaken DNA coding.

Make a commitment to a vision for your life from this day forward! This is a practice of Awakening. A daily, lifelong practice.

Exercise:

1. Write an I AM statement you will use. Make sure it is something you connect with. See examples below. It can be anything you choose.

Examples: I AM Powerful. I AM Limitless. I AM Divine Intelligence. I AM the Creator of My Life. (For more examples, see chapter 12.)

2. Create an Avatar to connect to your I AM.

Creating an Avatar:

The I AM creates a new identity which holds a higher Frequency than the programs that held space prior. This allows the *"environment"* of the cells to vibrate at a higher Frequency and invites the body to do so as well. The cells hold the new identity which enables you to do so.

Identity is the reason most people do not change. They cannot identify who they are beyond the reality they have created and identified within. When the body holds the Frequency pattern of the I AM, the new identity, it projects this Frequency into its environment. This shifts the way you think, feel and see the world around you. You actively use the I AM identity to give the conscious mind something to become.

Example: I Am Powerful:

Bring the Frequency of "I AM Powerful" into the expression of Pure Source Intelligence. You are setting the Avatar into an Intelligence beyond programmed reality.

This identity creates a very specific Frequency that creates a persona or Avatar that it is expressed through:

- Who are you if you are powerful?
- What are you choosing throughout the day?
- How are you thinking? How are you feeling?

Ask yourself these questions when you find yourself wanting to play small:

- If I AM Powerful, would I be playing small?
- Would I shy away from my own brilliance?

Create an Avatar around your I AM Statement:

- What do you look like if you are powerful?
- What are you wearing?
- How do you speak, connect to others?
- What are you doing with your life that is different from your experience up to now?

- **Consciously identify with your Avatar. Soon you meet the Frequency of your I AM and it becomes who you are! You no longer require Consciousness to become powerful. You are powerful!**

Become your Avatar. Merge with your new Frequencies:

- **Who am I as the Advanced Human?**
- **What do I look like? Allow the Intelligence to show you.**
- **What does it feel like to be an Advanced Human?**

Let your body attune to the Intelligence of the New Human. Notice how you feel and what you are thinking. Take a moment to create an Avatar of your NEXT. Who are you BECOMING?

Let the image come into your mind's eye. Once you see, hear, feel and know your Avatar, allow the person you are now to merge into the Avatar. The Avatar holds the Frequency of the new identity and shifts every cell of your body to become this new expression. Stay in the experience as you become your Avatar. Let yourself fully attune. Know you have the ability to self-actualize as your Avatar right now!

Take in one more deep breath. As you breathe out, know you are powerful enough to create beyond programmed reality. You are the Way.

Why are you committing to upgrading your human potential? Make sure you write out your **WHY** so you can reference it.

Complete your process with, **"Thank You. I Love You. It is done."**

State your I AM Statement aloud three times.

For the next three days, repeat this Evolution Technology activation. As you move throughout your day, be aware when you shift out of your I AM Avatar and into the loops of programmed reality.

Is Aging a Disease of Consciousness?

Using the mind to break looping cycles of the Matrix relies on the programming of your brain to create outcomes. Aging is a disease. You have been conditioned to believe you must age and deteriorate. This is not in alignment with what it is to be the Ascended Human. To advance beyond limitations of the mind, you must move into the Consciousness of the body. This is the next stage in human evolution.

You are a Creator Being through an Intelligence stored within the DNA. When you attune to this Intelligence with awareness, you shift out of the looping cycle of age and disease. To move out of the unconsciousness of cellular looping, you use awareness and become conscious of the Intelligence within your body.

The evolution of humanity is to use Consciousness to attune to the Intelligence of transcribed coding, bring cellular existence into a state of expression and break all looping cycles. You become the manifestation of the Ascended Human.

You are made of Pure Source Energy. You have the ability to bring this energy into no space and no time. You have been programmed that you will age through timelines held within the Matrix. How many times have you heard, "As you get older, things just start shutting down?"

To sustain and enhance the physical body as an evolved human is to become aware of thoughts held in programming and bring them into harmony held within the body's Intelligence. You are invited to live your life in the Frequency that your body, mind, and spirit are Divinely intended to be.

Any disease, including aging, is the breakdown of a perfectly created vessel for your Soul. You have the ability to live a life of awareness and reprogram your cells through DNA Coding.

There is an Infinite Source of life force energy within your physical body which holds information able to create longevity and vitality as a way of life. You can live within this state of Consciousness with practice.

It is your birthright to actively participate in the Ascension of the body and break the loop of age and disease. You can become conscious of your mind and body, allow your cells to respond in pure love and diminish disease, illness, and aging!

It is a choice! Choose new thoughts in each moment. New beliefs can be accessed each time you perceive yourself as a Creator.

D: Dream:

Claim your ability to consciously create 100% potential through attuning to your DNA Intelligence. Focus on the Frequency. Step into your Avatar to discover your possibility! You are already 100% potential. It is time to experience it!

Select something you wish to create as the New Human. This vision will be used to break from limited programming or looping cycles. Spend some time on what you desire to create. Dream Big!

Over the next few days, continue to connect to your Avatar. Challenge yourself to make choices from a higher Frequency than from where you have existed up to now. Become aware of where you are making choices from.

Break out of old thought patterns that come up. Bring awareness back to your dream and attune to the Intelligence your Avatar holds through pure Source Intelligence. In order to create as your Highest Potential, you must become aware of the looping patterns and create from choice. Awareness and choice are the pathways to upgrading human potential.

AWARENESS TOOL:

1. Identify where you feel you don't have a choice in your life. Where are you feeling stuck in a looping cycle?

Ask yourself, "Is this true?" Your first step is to take back your power and create choice. Even if it is something you cannot change, you can alter your perspective or experience of it.

2. What would it feel like to change or shift the frequency of these areas of your life?

3. Write about your Dream and what it looks like. Paint your dream in your mind and write it down. How do you look? How do you feel? How are you dressed? What does your hair look like? Look at yourself

in the mirror. See yourself as your Avatar living in your highest potential right now. What do you see, feel, sense? Dream Big!!

Exercise:

For the next 3 days:

1. Use the Evolution Technology to shift out of looping cycles you become aware of. Stay focused on your Dream as your Avatar.

2. State your I AM statement through the Frequency of your Avatar or the 3rd Symbol, **Scalar 33**, when you need an extra boost to break through old patterns.

3. If you are feeling stuck and can't see things clearly, close your eyes and say, **"Show me."** In this moment DNA intelligence attunes your body to the highest Frequency. Use your Intuitive Powers to read what is being shown.

4. In your mind's eye see DNA Codes activate in your body, leading you to 100% Potential. Play and discover just how powerful you are!

Learning the In and Out of Receiving or Expressing Energy

We may think, "I know my body can heal instantly but why does it take such a long time to see it heal?" This can also be related to losing weight, creating abundance or reversing aging.

The next step in absorbing the process is knowing that if you think, "I want to heal," it is the body that is expressing, and the body is healed.

Elevating and coding cellular memory is allowing something you "think" to be expressed in the body.

The thought is awakening the DNA Code holding the Frequency of the "answer to the thought." The Frequency has always been there; you are attuning to the specific Code that has the information through pure Source Intelligence. You will receive the answer from beyond programmed reality.

If you have the experience of expansion, it is an experience of Consciousness attuning to a higher Frequency. Evolution Technology allows your body to experience DNA Intelligence.

Your body is doing the "thinking," not your mind. ***Thinking is the thoughts beyond the programming of your mind.*** Your body becomes Divine Mind.

D: Dive Deep:

Think of something in your life you are struggling with. What feelings do you have about it? Bring this struggle to your awareness and notice how it affects your life, your thoughts and feelings.

As you go through your day, become aware of fears and triggers that elicit strong or negative thoughts. Do you hold back or become small because you are afraid of failure or being humiliated? Fear drains your life force energy.

It's important to notice when your energy drops. Every time your energy lowers over the next few days, put a mark on a piece of paper or in the notes of your phone. Write down what happened and what emotion was the strongest. Some examples are fear of not being heard, fear of not being accepted and fear of bringing attention to yourself.

Remember to be the observer. Do not judge yourself for your fears and feelings that arise. Just observe and record. Notice that when you observe, you are viewing through programmed reality. Notice when your Frequency shifts. This is the most important part of this exercise.

Exercise for the next 3 days:

1. Before you go to bed, review your list of observations from the day.

2. Recall situations when you felt your energy drop or when you were triggered.

3. Put a picture, an object, or a color to the first mark on your list in your mind's eye.

4. Use Evolution Technology to shift the Frequency of the picture, object or color you selected. Bring in the **Lu**, watch it spin and bring things to **Zero Point**. Follow with the **Sca**.

5. When bringing in the 3rd symbol, send love from your heart to the object.

6. Notice the Frequency shift. It is this easy to bring things into the expression of Source Intelligence!

7. Take a moment to attune your Consciousness to the DNA Codes that have been released. What information is there for you? Use your Intuitive Powers.

8. Repeat this exercise with all the marks on your list.

Rest! You are now living through the Intelligence of Source Frequency! Feel the power of the energy as it attunes your mind, body and spirit.

Regeneration: Life Extension

Cellular regeneration is the body's ability to recreate itself over and over. According to 3rd dimension programming, as you age, declining levels of stem cells affect a cell's ability to divide in perfect form. Your body depends on these "adult" stem cells in order to keep you healthy and to repair damage of any kind, such as from injury or illness.

Adult stem cells, one of the most important health discoveries of modern times, are critical to health and disease prevention. An age of stem cell therapy developments, including anti-aging treatments, followed this discovery.

Adult stem cells are created in the bone marrow. You are programmed to believe that the production of stem cells begins to decline as you age. When your levels of adult stem cells decline, damaged cells can be left unrepaired anywhere in the body, including the skin.

As a survival mechanism, the body will use what energy it has to repair the most vital organs. This means the repair of aging skin and hair may decline.

The "story" continues. Generally, by 35 years of age, stem cell production diminishes by 45 percent; by 50 years of age, by 50 percent and by 65 years of age, production diminishes by 90 percent! An infant's stem cells circulate at 100%. By age 65, stem cells are likely to have declined to 10% of their former potential.

As you step into the Ascended Human, you have the ability to shift this looping cycle! Evolution Technology offers the body the ability to regenerate cells to a Frequency beyond the looping cycle of cell division. You give the body what it needs to awaken Source Intelligence. Regeneration is something the body already knows. You are just elevating this ability to a super power level.

I: Imagine:

See yourself achieving your dream. Imagine yourself as your Avatar. See yourself exceeding beyond your wildest dreams. Imagine living a life of magic. Know you are a creation of Pure Source Intelligence.

Step into your Avatar. Imagine yourself achieving the highest level of human potential on a cellular level. What does your body feel like? What do you look like? How do you wake up in the morning? If you notice you have lowered your frequency, claim your ability to uplift your vibration.

Do you see yourself waking up and doing yoga before having tea and watching the sunrise? Do you go dancing or hiking? Visualize and feel yourself in these activities. Feel your body energized and full of life force energy. Keep the energy positive and exciting.

Your mind cannot tell the difference between dreaming an experience versus actually experiencing the same situation. The same parts of your brain light up and tell your body this is happening! The use of imagination is the first step to existing outside your programming. The more you imagine yourself in this elevated state, the more your body will rewire itself to this reality and become the New Human. Imagine! Imagine!

Exercise for the next 3 days:

Create your day through imagination! Pick one experience from your dream as the NEW Human and bring it into your life today. If you can't go dancing, dance around the house. If there is nowhere to hike, take a long walk. Improvise! Live your dream now!

Investigating Attachments to the Super Hologram

If you are going outside yourself to pull an energy into your experience, to create change, you are in "reflection" or "observation." You are creating within the Matrix or Super Hologram. Reflection of reality pulls information from the environment, outside yourself, in order to create.

When you create from the expression of the DNA, you are in "creation" of the Codes through Source Intelligence. At this point, you are projecting the expression out from the DNA's Divinity Codes and do not need to go outside into your environment to create a change in the expression of the DNA. The change is made within the Expression of Source moving from no space and no time beyond the Double Helix.

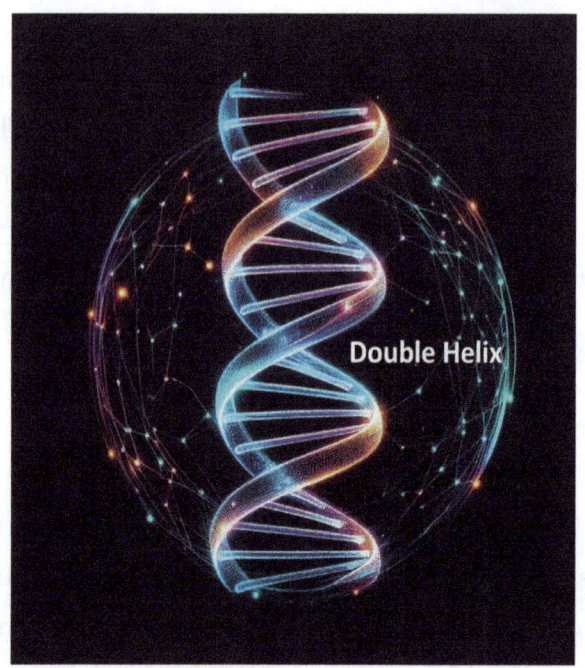

When you do these enough times, you realize that you can change expression of the DNA from within the DNA itself. You become the creator of the NEW Human. When in expression of the Intelligence holding information stored in the DNA, you create change in what it is to be human.

I: Investigate:

Live from your dream today in the expression of pure Source Intelligence! What thoughts do you have when you live in the mindset of expression? As you move throughout your day, notice when you begin to hook into your reality to find answers.

Take a moment to notice what Level of Consciousness you are viewing life from. Shift into the 4th Level of Consciousness. Listen and Do! Notice how you feel different. Bring Consciousness into your DNA and attune to the Intelligence there. Continue doing this every time you become aware of meeting your reality in the frequency it holds. Use the "1 to the 2 to the 3 to the 1" process in Chapter 13 to attune Consciousness to your experience beyond programmed reality.

Can you maintain thoughts through expression? Bring in the 3rd Symbol of the Evolution Technology, the **Scalar 33**. Place the Symbol around your body and picture a spiral expanding out from your DNA. As it moves through the 3rd Symbol, move all thought into Telethought and become DNA Intelligence.

Exercise for the next 3 days:

1. Each day write about a time you felt you hooked into the Super Hologram to receive energy and a time you were able to receive energy through the expression of DNA Intelligence.

2. Notice throughout the day moments when you had feelings or thoughts from programming. Break the pattern! Allow yourself to be uncomfortable not knowing what to do or how to feel. Let yourself be in the Unknown by not returning to your old thoughts and actions. Keep choosing to look forward. Use Evolution and DMT™ Technologies to shift and create focus through expression of DNA Intelligence.

3. Do an exercise each day that gives you life force energy. Even just 5 minutes will increase your Frequency.

You are made of energy. Life force is critical to your wellbeing. Life force allows you to experience life in fulfillment; without it you wouldn't be alive. When you feel ungrounded, lethargic, depressed or uncertain, you lose life force energy. When you integrate higher Consciousness and use intention, you feel empowered! You access higher states of mental and emotional energy that revitalize your physical and subtle bodies.

Here are some ways you can increase your life force energy:
- Be in nature
- Eat healthy life-giving foods
- Sleep
- Meditation
- Breathe
- Exercise
- Laugh
- Love

What makes you feel full of life?

Go do it!

Pick one of the above or choose another life affirming exercise to do each day. Take time to reconnect to the Bio-Life Intelligence within you and let it fully express itself in your reality!

Dissolving the Virus

A virus is a thought or program you live by unconsciously or are only slightly aware of. When you live life unconsciously, these viruses shape your reality. The patterns expand out from your mind, DNA or programmed frequency patterns into your energy system and into the world as you imagine it to be. All of it is filtered through your experience!

Aging is a disease prominent in Consciousness held in the looping cycle of the Super Hologram. Death is a disease of Consciousness. A repeated thought pattern that has been agreed upon through observation of the Matrix! A virus that is validated as you age because you unconsciously adapt to a belief system of the collective, parents, friends and teachers.

What you witness as your "reality" is constructed as you "see" through eyes that create your experience. What if it is not the truth? An aging body is just a symptom of a belief system or virus. This is a choice humanity continues to elect in the illusion of the Super Hologram!

How do you overcome a reality that has been passed down throughout the existence of mankind? First, you become conscious that reality is a reflection of the Consciousness you are holding. It is an energetic pattern that, just like a virus, extends from your body as a holographic reality. You have the ability to dissolve the virus by bringing it to the forefront of your mind and reprogram it into a more evolved energetic pattern through DNA Intelligence.

New energetic patterns are created when you repeatedly intercept old patterns. As unconscious thoughts come into your awareness, you acknowledge them, witness them and "choose" to no longer agree with them. Then you awaken Pure Source Intelligence through Evolution and DMT™ Technologies and replace them with the expression of Pure Source Intelligence. You break the loop all together. You "upgrade" Human Potential.

An "upgrade" occurs when you replace dense energy patterns, viruses or slow moving particles and shift them to a higher spin state which holds Pure DNA Intelligence. This is something your mind cannot register because it hasn't yet had the experience. Your eyes cannot see it at its purest Frequency. Your body cannot register it consciously because you have not experienced it.

Ask for it to move into expression. Using Evolution Technology, request to be upgraded to the New Human. A human that is not limited by thought patterns of the Super Hologram! Become the Ascended or Evolved Human and create from the Unknown. A new reality is inviting you to consciously join it! You use this process until you become Pure Source Intelligence.

You have everything you need to dissolve the laws of the Matrix. Use awareness and choice to challenge your mind to shift beyond observation of the illusion itself. When the programs or viruses of the collective creep into your awareness, use the Technologies to dissolve the illusion!

Be a Consciousness advocate. Push the bounds of what seems possible. Find your inspirations through the impossible. Most say you must inevitably abide by the laws of the Universe. Start to question this reality. Decide today how you want to **"Gamify Reality"** through the awakening of Pure Intelligence where law does not exist because it is of Pure Essence where law is not needed.

V: VIRUS:

What virus are you holding within your Dream? A virus is a program that you live by without being conscious of it. You are unaware that you are stuck in its loop. When you live within the looping pattern of the illusion, you have no control over your life or any outcome.

Pick one virus you feel you are "infected" with. Locate that underlying feeling you have deep down inside that is usually stronger when in stressful situations. When creating the New Human, though it is a positive thing, your body registers it as change and finds the shift stressful. Your body resists change and runs viruses so that you feel "safe," both unconsciously and consciously.

Change is challenging because your body is chemically wired to resist it so as to keep things the same. This will be your experience even if your current state is keeping you unhealthy, tired and unhappy. The body doesn't distinguish between "good" or "bad" change. It registers the shift as stress and releases chemicals to resist it. These chemicals trigger your viruses.

Examples of Viruses:

- I am not good enough.
- I will fail.
- I don't know what I'm doing.
- I'm not healthy enough to do what I want.
- I'm too old to learn something new, to reverse aging.
- This is impossible.
- Anything agreed upon through observation of the Super Hologram.

Exercise:

1. Write down a few of your viruses. Now look at the list and pick the one that has the most charge or effect on your happiness.

2. Throughout the next three days, notice when your virus interferes with your creation. Just notice it. Look it straight in the eye. Keep observing yourself as the virus comes up. Is it spreading? How does it feel? Once you have seen it clearly, use the Technologies to activate DNA Intelligence.

3. First use Evolution Technology to shift the pattern, then DMT™ Technology to hold focus in Telethought as the Intelligence.

4. You may still feel, act out, and continue the pattern but you will do it consciously. This is the first step to breaking the pattern! The next time you see or feel your virus come up, observe again. Repeat the Technologies. Explore the virus through the Intelligence. Start to notice how it is different.

Celebrate that every time you observe a virus, you are Upgrading your Human Potential. You are becoming the Ascended Human.

Living a High Frequency Life:

Living a life at high Frequency requires that you be aware of thoughts that are not in line with your truth. To live in awareness is to create choice.

Jewels' Story:

"Over 30 years ago when I started working as a vibrational practitioner, I instantly noticed a difference in how I felt. I felt connected and at peace with the world around me. Being around Frequency work opened my eyes to a world of vibration. I started

studying what energy is on a Quantum level and how it could be used to shift how I identified in the 3D world."

So how does it work? And how can you take it to the next level? You are made of energy. Within your body you have places where energy vibrates in a high spin state which creates balance and health. When illness, injury, or depression are present, it indicates a lack of energy and a low spin state.

In the physics realm, energy is a property of objects which can be transferred to other objects or converted into different forms. Thus, you can shift form by transferring slow moving particles to higher spin rates.

How can you use this understanding of energy to reach 100% Human Potential? If you are made of energy, then it is possible to convert or change your form using energy. All energy has a frequency at which it vibrates. For instance, a magazine has particles that are very close together making it have more solid form or low frequency. The emotion of shame is the frequency of about 20 Hz. The emotion of peace is around 600 Hz.

When thoughts and emotions are in the Frequency of peace, you vibrate at a much higher rate. When you notice that some people seem to "glow" and others seem to have a cloud around them, you are picking up their frequency.

The higher the Frequency, the better you feel. The energy at which you are vibrating is reflected in how you show up, your health and your overall wellbeing.

When receiving higher Frequencies, such as through Evolution Technology, your body resonates in a higher state and a shift occurs in the energy of your body, mind and energy body. DNA intelligence, when activated into expression, will bring low vibrational particles, thought patterns and emotions into a higher Frequency. You then become the higher Frequency.

When the energy of your body reaches a high vibrational state, it remembers what it is like to exist in that Frequency and desires to remain there. In time Consciousness meets this Frequency, you self-actualize and hold the new state. How you view reality shifts.

In order for this to happen, your energy system "releases" lower vibrations that cannot resonate with the higher Frequency. These lower vibrational blocks are programs.

Most illnesses in the body start with a program, a thought or emotion connected to a story that plays out in daily life. This can be conscious or unconscious.

Clearing programs connected to anxiety, depression, anger, or shame brings a life of choice. In which vibration do you desire to live life? You have the power to bring in Divine Expression to create a life beyond the looping cycle of the Super Hologram!

Reprogramming the body and its responses can be done with practice and awareness. When you fall into a lower vibration of anxiety, anger, or such, you have a choice to interrupt the negative pattern. See it for what it is... a program! A program is a story you have come to live by that is not true. It is the Super Hologram.

A higher vibration is always available. As a conscious being, you have the power to be aware. You are energy. Energy will vibrate where it is directed consciously until you hold that energy in Pure Intelligence. You have the choice to live a life of freedom.

The world around you is a reflection of the frequency in which you resonate. Use the Matrix to shift your Frequency beyond it. Do things that raise your vibration such as eating healthy, exercising, meditating, drinking high Frequency water and receiving healing therapies. Use the tools you have to support your journey.

What do you want to create with your energy? If you resonate at a high vibration, you create a high Frequency life! You begin to **"Gamify Reality."** You have energy that flows through you and extends out into your surroundings.

Fields of energy around and within you are measurable forces in an information grid that connects you to all aspects of your health and wellbeing. This grid is still a part of the Super Hologram. It can be used consciously to see beyond the illusion of limitations you experience through it. The information stored in this grid, or energy system, connects you to all things. It is key to **Breaking the God Code/Breaking Quantum Physics**.

Socrates said, "Energy, or soul, is separate from matter and the Universe is made of energy – pure energy which was there before man and other material things like the Earth came along."

Quantum Physics says that as you go to the deeper workings of an atom, you find there is nothing there. It remains as just energy waves taking up space. An atom is actually an invisible force field, a kind of miniature tornado, which emits waves of electrical energy.

When using Evolution Technology to improve health and wellbeing, you receive direct Frequencies of DNA Intelligence. For example, if you are suffering from a cold, the Frequency of healthy blood cells and a strong immune system will begin to express through the Double Helix into the body so you can consciously attune to the Pure Essence of perfect form. Evolution Technology awakens an Intelligence within you that is in a vibration beyond the frequency of the Super Hologram.

What frequency do you vibrate at?

V: Validate:

Bring your attention to the vibration of your dream. Focus on the positive energy it holds and take the time to bring Consciousness into the Frequency. Attune to the Intelligence within it. Be grateful for the opportunity to experience an Intelligence beyond your programming. The more you see through the creation of your dream, the more you begin to experience the 4th and 5th Levels of Consciousness.

Exercise for the next 3 days:

1. Pick an I AM statement you can start to live by to replace your virus.

   Examples:

   - I AM an Alchemist.
   - I AM Divine Perfection.

- I Always Do My Best.
- I AM Impeccable.
- I AM Love.
- I AM the New Human.

2. Choose a small goal you wish to accomplish today.

3. Example: For the next three days, when I look in the mirror, I will see beyond the illusion of form.

4. As you go through your day, look for the reflection of your goal through the different layers of frequency. Can you see it through the illusion of the Super Hologram? Can you invite in the experience beyond it?

5. When you become aware of a virus creeping in, use Evolution Technology followed by the DMT™ Technology. Connect to your I AM and become the expression of the Intelligence beyond programmed reality. Practice.

Breaking Victim Mentality

Are you the victim of your life circumstances? Are you ready to be accountable for your life? To stay in awareness that everything is a choice?

You cannot ascend to a higher state of Consciousness if you are blaming, dumbing it down or trying to control. Are you compromised by Victim Mentality? Observe the Consciousness you hold when you resist life.

Your resistance can be seen as one of two choices, the other being empowerment. Both are available but are played out differently. One, resisting the Super Hologram and one, using the Hologram to awaken an Intelligence beyond. Victim Mentality is created anytime you "act out" resistance to what life, the Super Hologram, is showing you.

As you go through your week, become aware of how you react to stress in your life. Do you blame the situation? Do you pretend there is nothing wrong? Do you try to control it or others so that you feel okay or in control?

Upgrading your human potential isn't about having the perfect life; it's about identifying and holding a Frequency that resonates with your experience. It is having awareness of what you are creating with your thoughts and vibrations.

In this week's exercise, you will be the observer of the Super Hologram/Matrix to discover where you play the victim role. Every day, journal times that you discover yourself blaming, trying to control the outcome or tuning out/shutting down.

Remember, overdoing is another way of tuning out. Observe what other ways you avoid accountability, choice or use distraction to stay small or resist change.

Make a list of ways you dismiss your choice to see beyond the looping cycle and become a victim of your mind or circumstances. This is the first step to taking action. Use Evolution Technology to change your life. It is important to discover your patterns when being the victim.

Here is a list of ways the victim pattern can be played out:

- Blame, the number one expression of Victim Mentality
- Over stimulating yourself or over doing in order to avoid a feeling or situation
- Bringing others into conflict by needing to have someone on your side
- Repeating an experience verbally or mentally over and over without coming to a solution
- Control, either of the situation or people in the situation
- Playing the "poor me" role
- Manipulation
- Bullying
- Using passive aggressive behaviors to manipulate the situation
- Dumbing it down or pretending you don't understand when you do
- Shutting down or cutting yourself off

Add to the List! Victim mentality is anything you do consciously or unconsciously that is giving away your power. It allows outside circumstances to have control over how you feel, act or react.

When you identify the pattern, feel it in your body. Where is the energy being held? Is it leaking, burning, building density? Is your heartbeat racing?

Knowing when you are in a chemical response to a situation is key to Ascension. You become aware that you have a choice in an experience you normally react to.

It takes practice to override the body's response to stress. Because you are a conscious being, you always have a choice.

As you move into higher Frequencies and hold higher states of Consciousness, you may experience body sensations that feel uncomfortable. Learning to identify responses, and thought patterns that accompany them, is a huge step in moving past plateaus or stagnant energy.

When saying to yourself, "I just can't get past this" or "I can't seem to change this no matter what I do," or the big one, "I have been doing this work for 30 some years and I still am not where I want to be," then you know you have self-actualized in an energy and have not moved beyond it. You are invited to discover who you identify as and invite in a Frequency beyond it.

V: Victim:

Notice where you fall victim to your virus, your life or stagnant energy. Take back the power! When you are accountable for your thoughts, feelings, and actions, you create choice and empowerment.

When you blame others for your thoughts, feelings and actions, you lose your power to them and become a victim of your circumstances. It is always a choice to be accountable. Where in your life do you lose your power? Is it to a co-worker that gets under your skin? A relative you can't forgive? Your spouse or friend that just never understands?

Exercise for the next 3 days:

1. As you go throughout your day, be aware of when you become a victim. Is it a driver that cuts you off on your way to work? The store clerk that is rude for no reason? What thoughts come up? Do you blame, get angry or do you shut down? Start becoming aware of the story you tell yourself when you become the victim. Do you blame circumstances or people when your vibration drops?

2. Write out one experience either from today or from the past when you became the victim. Write out how you justified yourself and what you did.

    Did you tell others your story so you would have someone "on your side?" Did you get angry and attack? Did you get quiet and sad until someone asked you what was wrong so you could "tell your story" and get sympathy? Did you manipulate the other person into being wrong or bad?

Become aware of your energy cycle so you can awaken to the new Intelligence waiting to move into expression. Become aware of your victim patterns.

You can't live a life of pure essence and vitality, a life as the New Human, when you give your energy away to circumstances. When you become the victim, you look for ways to get energy from other places. This cycle is seen everywhere in your life if you really look. It is the looping cycle.

Some get angry to take energy from people; the other person gives energy by either fighting back, playing small or becoming the victim. This exchange of energy is an example of how loops get created. Break the looping cycle! Say "no" to Victim Mentality!

You are accountable for every part of your life. You have a choice. Notice when you become the victim and see what pattern you gravitate to most. Awakening calls for change. Change is the evolution of You!

The Awakening: You have a Choice:

Identifying when you are being a victim is the first step to becoming conscious of looping patterns. When you are unconscious, you live life in a state of mind where life happens to you. You are pulled into the drama of the Matrix and get sucked into the hamster wheel. You feel disconnected from your truth, feel alone and that you have no control over your life.

The day you choose to no longer be a victim is the day you "awaken." Yes, you may fall victim to certain circumstances again, but once awakened, you remember that you are the Creator and the Creation. When you move out of repeated patterns or the Super Hologram and begin attuning to DNA Intelligence, you step into a power that is beyond the illusion.

When you experience the Super Hologram/Matrix, you become aware of where you are vibrating. Loops ready to be broken are revealed. The Super Hologram shows you the frequency that matches your Consciousness. You judge an experience as good and bad when you filter through programming or the ego.

Observe an experience without meeting the frequency it holds. Invite in an Intelligence beyond it and notice if you are able to shift into a space beyond the illusion of what is seen. By doing so, you create an opportunity to have the experience in a state of Consciousness beyond the Super Hologram. Resistance is the need to hold onto an experience; it creates static energy and density. If you do not shift beyond resistance, you remain held in the illusion of the Matrix.

You lose life force energy when you resist life. When you move into higher states of Consciousness, you break the looping cycle. Trust in the Intelligence within you. Let go of the need to control and allow yourself to attune to the magic beyond the illusion itself. When you experience resistance, use it as an opportunity to grow to an even higher state of Consciousness. A state of being where you vibrate at and attract higher Frequency experiences!

Your telomeres and DNA have their own Intelligence. You reprogram your DNA to what it means to be a New Human by becoming conscious and letting go of resistance. This allows you to maintain life force energy. Celebrate the good and the uncomfortable because it is all communication; it gives you information to shift beyond the illusion! Enjoy the ride of your own evolution! Enter the Unknown and trust.

E: Exercise:

You may get stuck in negative emotions and self-talk. Choose to shift your energy! Using exercises to move through challenging mental, emotional and physical reactions help you stay empowered and not fall victim to life. When you feel triggered, use an exercise. Start with the Evolution Technology.

You may notice you have the same reaction pattern to a situation. For example, you have the same fight about the same thing with your husband. You worry every month about your weight or health and think the same things and feel the same way each time. These are patterns your body is addicted to and recreates over and over because it's what it knows. This is the looping cycle!

Here are some exercises that may be helpful to break chemical and mental patterns during stressful situations. Move into the Unknown by breaking the circuit. Use these tools to reprogram conscious and unconscious programs. Start creating from the Unknown by using the Evolution Technology, instead of "recreating" what you have done before. Use these tools to support the shift.

A Box of Tools:

1. **Count from 5 to 1...** 5 4 3 2 1. When you get to one you must "DO" something. This tells your mind to get out of the lower part of the brain where you get stuck in emotion and negativity and to move to the conscious part of the brain where you make choices!

   It is best to do something you have to "think" to do. Go upstairs and wash your hands in a sink you never use. Rearrange the towels in the closet. Keep going until you are thinking clearly and can use the Evolution Technology to shift you into a higher spin state.

2. **Experience:** Choose to be your I AM statement and "DO" something such as breathe deeply, journal, dance for five minutes, become the observer or "shake it off" with your

hands. If all else fails, start naming what you are experiencing: "My heart rate is elevated." "My hands are sweating." "I feel sad and angry." "It hurts in my heart." "My breathing is shallow, and it hurts to move."

Naming what you are experiencing makes you more conscious of what is actually happening and keeps you away from being lost in the story and allowing the virus to take over.

3. **Breathe!** Take a deep breath and refocus. Focusing on the breath makes it hard to focus on your negative thoughts. This is a great one to do when you are driving, working or in public.

4. **Reset!** Tell yourself to "RESET." Reset to your intention. Become your Avatar. Remind yourself it's okay to make a mistake, that it's how you handle it that matters.

Do you become the victim of your virus and spread it to others, or do you use it to fuel your conscious choice to become the Creator of your life? This is a choice you make over and over and over!

"RESET" is telling your brain to not move into a habit or response and gives you the signal to consciously choose to do it differently! New experiences are the way your body will change reactive responses. Remind yourself of your goal and focus through the Evolution and DMT™ Technologies.

Now come up with an exercise you feel would work for you! Remember that an exercise is just that. You do it over and over just like learning a new sport or language. It is a practice of Consciousness. Just like a muscle, the more you do it, the more it will work until it becomes natural.

Training yourself to be the one that is in control of your reaction to the Super Hologram is a lifelong commitment. It is the commitment that makes you either a Creator or a Victim. You always have this choice!

Exercise:

For the next 3 days:

1. Pick one or a couple of the tools above.

2. When you feel stuck or reactive, use the tools. Write down how it feels when you do them. Did you learn something about yourself? How easy or hard was it to move into empowerment? Did you discover a new virus?

Now notice how the tools are enhanced when you add the Technologies. Take time to shift and attune your Consciousness to the awakening of Source Intelligence. Explore the information stored there. Focus comes through Telethought, Thought through DNA Intelligence.

E: Elevate:

Increase the energy or vibration of your life to meet the highest level of Intelligence you can hold. Your life is a vibrational match to the Frequency your DNA is expressing and the Consciousness held there.

You create a New Human reality when you choose to attune to DNA Intelligence and unhook from the Matrix. Can you feel the Frequency shift when using Evolution Technology? Are you taking time to consciously attune to the shift? Notice how long you can hold Consciousness in the Divine Expression that is activated.

Elevate your vibration by consciously attuning to the Frequencies that release when practicing the Technologies. Be your best cheerleader! Celebrate when you self-actualize in higher Frequencies. The journey is fun!

Exercise:

1. Take some time today to consciously attune to Frequencies activated when using the Evolution Technology.

2. Connect to the Frequency with your Avatar. Is it different now?

3. Play! Keep exploring the Technology and where to bring it into your life for better focus and strength. What limitations can you bypass where you were stuck before?

Awareness is Awakening! New experiences are the way your body changes reactive responses. Remind yourself of your Dream and self-discover in the Frequency it holds. Allow the New Human to emerge in everything you do. Make new choices when you are faced with thoughts that are of the Matrix. Remember, the brain cannot tell the difference between an actual experience and an imagined experience.

When you imagine and feel a new experience, you are firing new responses just by thinking and feeling it is true! Be aware of old patterns and use Evolution Technology to shift back into Divine Expression.

Living in Eternity: The Flower of Life is the Inversion or the Matrix

You are more than you "think" you are. When you identify in Frequency, know that until you become 100% potential, it is only part of the truth. Your mind filters out what is conceived as "not useful" in every moment because it can only be conscious of focused thought in a linear or non-spatial timeline. When using Intuitive Powers, you have the ability to use Telethought, be aware of spherical time and hold focus in many timelines or many waves of information at one time.

You currently use only 10% of your brain and DNA Intelligence. So much of your reality is unseen. The dormant part of your brain holds a vast amount of information available to you. In essence, it is the purest part of you.

Frequency patterns that hold information and vibrations that attain knowledge, wisdom, and a power beyond your conscious understanding are waiting to be "turned on." You can use Consciousness as a tool to become this Intelligence.

Your Intuitive Powers are a state of being. In the most advanced state, you no longer think, sense, hear or know things through observation. The "Listen and Do" becomes just "Do." You become Source Intelligence. This is 100% Human Potential as understood at this moment.

DNA is an energy held in expression, bypassing observation. It connects you to the Intelligence held there. You have the ability to experience Oneness. Oneness is Pure Essence, meaning it is not in a state of observation.

You begin to colonize your surroundings by connecting to Pure Intelligence and become your environment. If you were to see this Intelligence as energy, it would look like connective tissue.

It connects all that is. It connects you to every dimension and goes beyond space and time. This energy is the foundation of life outside the looping system. It can only be accessed through the expression of DNA Intelligence.

The Matrix or Super Hologram can be used as a reflection of Divine Intelligence until you move beyond Consciousness held in observation. Moving beyond the limitation of the physical world, know that this energy is your truest essence. You have the ability to use it to expand your life beyond limiting beliefs, illnesses, thoughts or anything that holds you back from being your fullest potential!

DNA or Source Intelligence is where you grow into the highest version of yourself! Within this Intelligence you ascend into a human capable of being 100% potential. This is who you were born to be! This capability is just waiting dormant within you, ready to be ignited. DNA is a gateway to life beyond what you know or understand. It is not understood by Science and is not within the Quantum Field. It has no limitation and will break the looping cycle of age and disease.

Explore and experience life beyond what is physical. Your physical makeup is just an energy pattern waiting to be "upgraded." You begin to upgrade what it means to be human by experiencing life in the uncomfortable.

It may seem crazy to think you can live an Eternal Life. Yet, it makes no sense to repeat what has been done before…over and over. Humans evolve. The next step is to go where no man has gone. Change your world by changing yourself. Upgrade what it means to be human by allowing the unseen to be expressed through DNA Intelligence.

E: Emerge and Execute:

Become aware of your thoughts and emotions throughout your day. Such awareness opens opportunities to see beyond what is seen. Once you see a pattern, use Evolution Technology to shift into an experience through Source Intelligence. Have fun and explore what information you intuitively connect to when doing this.

Awareness offers choice. Practice being the Creator and the Creation of the New Human in all areas of your life. The more you "practice" being the Creator, the more natural it will become and the more you tap into Consciousness beyond what you are currently holding. You attune to Source Intelligence just by using the Technology on a daily basis and being conscious of the information held within it.

Exercise:

Keep going! Make it a daily practice to use the Evolution and DMT™ Technologies. Notice when you fall into old thought patterns and emotional responses and explore what new experiences open up when you continue "turning on" DNA Intelligence.

Keep going deeper! The more you awaken, the more you create your highest potential. The more you live your life at your highest potential, the more empowered you become. The more empowered you become, the more you become Source Intelligence! You have the ability to live in the Consciousness of this Intelligence until you become the Intelligence.

Daily Exercise:

Write out one time you were able to notice an old pattern and break it. How did you do it? How did it feel? Be grateful! Evolution Technology is a Consciousness tool! Make it a practice every morning and night by exploring what it is capable of igniting within you. Use the Technology and explore where you can overcome limitations.

When you feel you are losing focus, tap into the Technology. Notice that your ability to stay focused increases with practice. See that, by igniting the Technology when exerting yourself, you can achieve much more! Bypass the laws of the Universe through the Intelligence stored within you.

Continue practicing the Evolution and DMT™ Technologies and discover how long you can hold Consciousness in a state of expression. Keep practicing and exploring beyond the limitations of the Super Hologram. See yourself becoming 100% Human Potential!

Notes

Notes

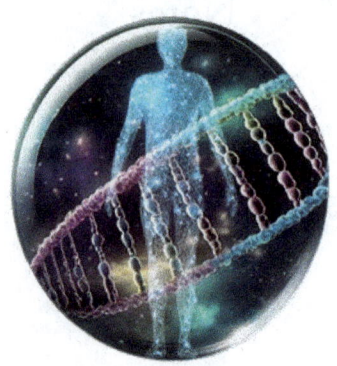

Chapter 18: Upgrading Human Potential Through Body Chemistry: 6 Day Challenge

- **Day 1: Set your intention.**

- **Day 2: Serotonin**: Maximize cognitive function and move beyond the limitations of the mind.

- **Day 3: Dopamine**: Use the Frequency of Dopamine for motivation, inspiration and open pathways of an internal energy propelling you into the highest version of self in creation of the next step of your intention.

- **Day 4: Oxytocin**: Open to clear communication with your inner guidance and cut out all chatter to create your best life. Express self-love from an internal knowing of who you are at a Soul level.

- **Day 5: Lactate/Endorphins**: Become aware of how you view the limitations of your body and activate an Intelligence that brings you to the next level of performance.

- **Day 6: DMT™**: Experience a DMT™ activation that shifts cellular function into higher spin rates or Frequency waves, allowing the body to shift out of disease and deterioration.

Day One:
Set Your Intention and Create an Avatar

Today, you set your intention on **WHAT** you will focus on to master the highest potential of your body. This allows you to tap into an energy beyond what you previously have experienced. Your intention is the focal point you will use to practice and experience the Intelligence. This is your body at optimal performance!

WHAT is the challenge? The challenge you will master over the next 6 days is the part of you that keeps you stuck in the loop of how your body performs currently. You are stuck in the chemical makeup of the body.

These chemicals control your experiences emotionally, physically, cognitively and create your experience of overall wellbeing. You have the ability to become an Intelligence beyond the experience of the body as it is now.

When setting your intention, your **WHAT**, take a moment to ask yourself **WHY**? From where are you asking for this shift? Are you looking to fulfill an emotion? To be happier? To feel safe? For freedom? Be aware of what emotion your body is asking for. This will be important information for your journey. What emotion is being fulfilled by your intention?

Today sit with your intention and notice how, by just calling it in, you begin to focus on it. Your intention has a Frequency, and this Frequency has an Intelligence.

As you go throughout your day, notice where you are focusing your attention. Are you looking at your intention from the you who you are now or are you looking at it from the person that is experiencing creation of the intention?

Your challenge today is to focus on your intention, to know what emotion you are looking to fulfill with your intention and to notice who is focusing on the practice itself.

Can you focus as the person who is in creation of the intention? As the person experiencing the intention? Or are you focusing on the intention from who you are right now?

Write out your intention, your emotion that you are looking to fulfill and describe the person you are if you live in the highest potential of your intention.

> **What are you feeling?**
> **What do you do with your day?**
> **What thoughts are you thinking?**
> **How do you dress, speak and connect with others?**

We will see you tomorrow! It is time to **Bio-Hack Energy** and **Live your Optimal Life!**

Day Two:
Upgrading Serotonin

Today you tap into the Intelligence of the **FREQUENCY** of Serotonin. How does Serotonin make you feel?

Serotonin is a chemical messenger that acts as a mood stabilizer. It helps with good sleeping patterns as well as to boost your mood. Research shows that Serotonin levels can have an effect on mood and behavior.

The chemical is commonly linked to feeling good and living longer. Use the Intelligence of the Frequency of Serotonin to maximize cognitive function and move beyond the limitations of the mind.

Today you will learn to choose and act beyond your emotional response when "thinking" something will make you happy. When you are thinking something will make you happy, you are most often thinking through programming. You are searching for an emotional sensation instead of creating from a clear state of Frequency or being.

When you activate the Frequency of Serotonin versus the chemical release of Serotonin, the body resonates in an Intelligence which allows you to make decisions beyond personal programming and collective consciousness.

Bring focus to your intention. Are you searching and making choices through the chemical of Serotonin which is created through programmed responses? Instead, boost your ability to create choices from Pure Intelligence!

Serotonin Challenge:

Make a choice or do something today through the Frequency of Serotonin. Do the activation and sense the difference between the Frequency of Serotonin with its Intelligence versus the chemical of Serotonin. You will notice the difference.

The Frequency is cleaner, clearer and doesn't fluctuate depending on what you experience outside this Frequency. This is an example of who you are becoming beyond the looping cycle of the body.

This is the body's Intelligence beyond programmed reality. Today, begin to make choices from a place of pure focus through the Frequency of Serotonin. Notice how much clearer your thoughts are, how easy choices are made and how focused you can be within the choice itself.

Day Three:
Dopamine

Dopamine is released when you expect a reward or a fix. You may associate a certain activity with pleasure. Just the thought of the activity or substance, for example, a certain food, sex or shopping, can be enough to raise Dopamine levels.

Dependence on a chemical response of the body to create habits that feel rewarding can create loops that do not serve your best interests. Your body can become addicted to the chemical of Dopamine and search for a quick fix.

Today you will use the **FREQUENCY** of Dopamine for motivation and inspiration…to open pathways and release an internal energy to propel you to the highest version of yourself. From here you create your intention.

Create from the Frequency of Dopamine when looking for a quick fix, reward or motivation. Use the Frequency to retain focus to achieve your goal. Remain in the Frequency and continue to connect it to your intention even when it gets uncomfortable.

A quick fix could be to quit, cheat, or take an easier route. Shift it! Using the Frequency of Dopamine holds your body in a clean energy that propels you into Creation as the Creator. Continue to tap into the Frequency of Dopamine.

Day 3 Challenge:

Tapping into the Frequency of Dopamine, take an Inspired Action from your clear choices from Day 2.

Day 4:
Oxytocin

Oxytocin is a natural hormone that stimulates the "Falling In Love Effect." One purpose is the continuation of mankind through primal response.

The ascended state of Oxytocin, the **FREQUENCY**, can be used to create clear communication with your inner knowing or guidance. It facilitates the removal of all mind chatter and allows you to stay in creation as your best self. Self-love is expressed as an internal knowing of who you are at a Soul level.

You show up as your best self when falling in love. You discover yourself anew. View yourself through the Frequency of self-love. As the Frequency of Oxytocin is met, it attunes Consciousness to Pure Intelligence.

Clear communication reveals itself when in a Frequency beyond programming. Notice the absence of mind chatter. Revel at the guidance that comes when you open yourself up to the possibilities.

Use the Frequency of love to discover through imagination, guidance and creative flow. A purity of guidance comes in when the chatter and self-doubt go away.

Feel the purest state of Oxytocin in your body when no chemicals are activated.

Sense how powerful you are when you use Frequency with focus and intention.

Day 4 Challenge:

The Ascended DMT™ Conscious Accelerator is sacred geometry. Use the Ascended DMT™ Conscious Accelerator to support focus:

- The shape itself holds a Technology that bypasses timelines and supports holding focus in the "now moment."

- Visualize yourself within the sphere of the Accelerator. From within the sphere, push your thoughts, connected to your intention, into the Pyramids. Feel your thoughts being held in the magnetic field.

- The Symbols allow thought to connect to DNA /Source Intelligence and bypass programmed reality.

- Notice how your thoughts change.

- The Pyramids create a magnetic field that holds Consciousness in expression of Higher Intelligence.

- This trains the mind to hold expression. To focus beyond programming.

- The sphere holds a Technology, creating space to shift from observing programmed reality to expressing Source Intelligence.

Advanced Use:

- Visualize yourself within the Sphere.

- Connect to the Ascended DNA Mitochondria Cell within the Pineal Gland. Ask for the specific Frequency you desire to access. See the DNA release this Frequency, expand from the Pineal Gland and push into the Pyramids.

- From within the Sphere, connect thought into the Pyramids. Feel thought being held in the magnetic field.

- Attune your thoughts within the magnetic field to DNA/Source Intelligence.

- Allow the Technology to support you in holding thought in expression of the specific Intelligence you are working with.

- Repeat as needed.

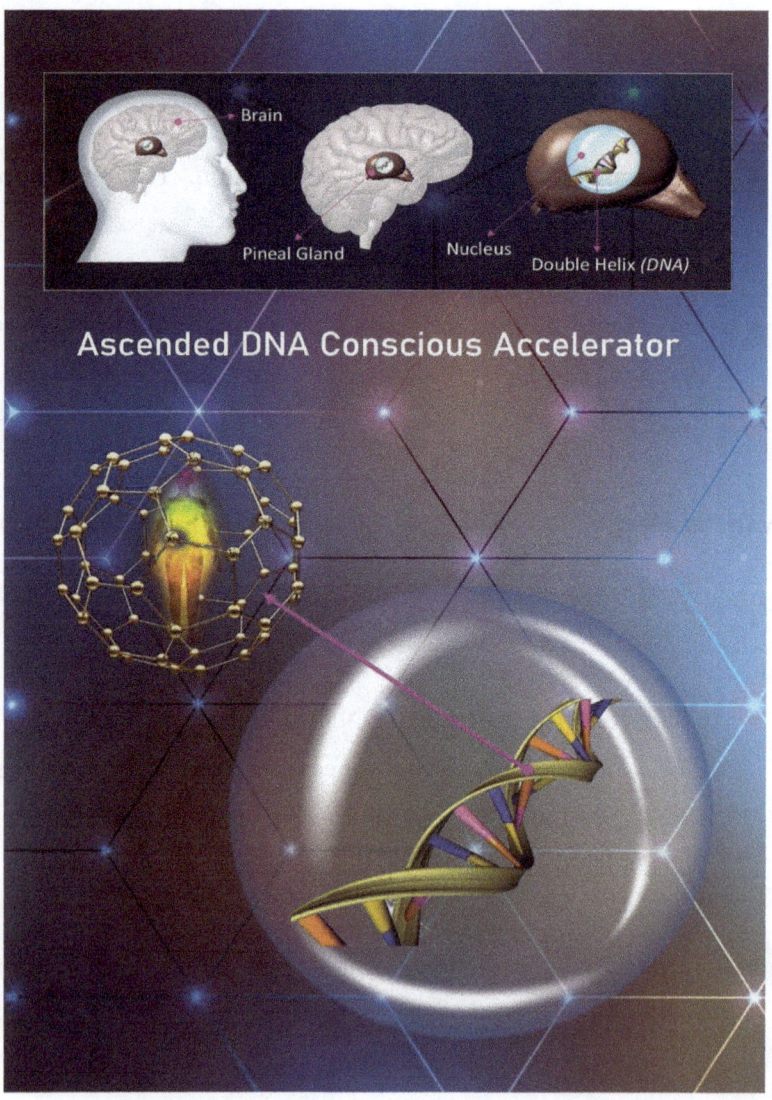

Day Five: Lactate and Endorphins

Become aware of how you view the limitations of your body. You have the ability to perform beyond limitations and activate an Intelligence that brings you to a higher level of performance.

Lactate is oxygen used during aerobic activities to produce energy. But when oxygen is limited, as when working out for long periods of time or weightlifting, the body runs low on oxygen and begins to pull on hydrogen. The body temporarily converts pyruvate into a substance called Lactate which allows glucose breakdown and energy production to continue.

Endorphins are the "runner's high," the amazing feeling you get after a great workout. Endorphins have many benefits to the body, including reduced pain and discomfort, better mood, improved self-esteem and increased pleasure.

When Endorphins release, you may experience inspired thoughts and solutions to life's situations. This is where the body meets the Frequency of Lactate which is connected to the Frequency of DMT™.

DMT™ is the chemical that brings insight beyond programmed reality. Today you will move into a state of high Frequency performance using the vibrational patterns of Lactate and Endorphins.

Maximize your workout with specific Frequency integration exercises!

Your body can easily keep going even when the mind says you cannot. There is no such thing as weakness or strength. Only those who use self or Spiritual Discipline will discover the power of Lactate.

The magic happens when you focus on who you are becoming and choose to continue even when you want to give up. It is much easier to do this when you use the Frequency of Lactate connected to DMT™.

Begin to keep track of your workouts. Notice when you practice adding Lactate/ DMT™, that your body can go longer, stronger and harder. See your body as the perfection it is meant to be as you move beyond primal responses and maximize the chemicals of your body as Intelligence. As you break through limitations, you begin to turn on the other 90% of your potential!

https://becomingbioquantum.com/enhanceperformance

Day Six:
DMT™

What is DMT and how can we use it? DMT is produced in the Pineal Gland. It is released when you are born and when you die. The Frequency of DMT™ holds your Soul's Essence and is encoded into the Ascended DNA.

When you die, the Codes move back into your Soul so that your purest essence is never lost. The truth is you do not need to die to tap into the Coding of your purest essence... you at 100% potential.

DMT™ has a very similar Frequency to Lactate. They work together to create a Field where the body turns on potential beyond the looping cycles of how you experience the body now.

DMT naturally occurs in small amounts in your brain, cerebrospinal fluid and other tissues of the body. You can connect to the Frequency of DMT™ and tap into an Intelligence beyond programming.
Today you will experience a DMT™ activation that shifts your focus and workout into a magnetic field of Frequency and allows you to bypass limitations and experience the body in optimal states of being.

Become the new version of you. Live beyond the chemical responses of the body and experience life in the Frequency of 100% human potential.

Chemicals are created to express your full potential. They hold a bridge of Consciousness to who and what you are beyond the chemical. Each chemical has an Intelligence. You are called to use Intelligence to maximize your potential to become the NEXT in human evolution!

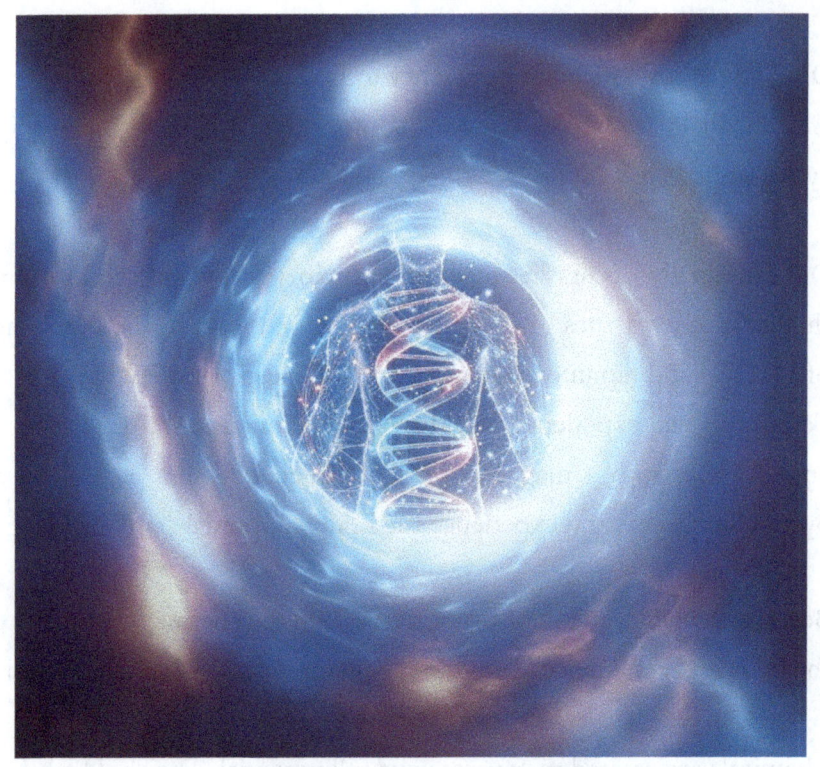

Maximize Performance with DMT™:

https://becomingbioquantum.com/MaximizePerformance

Tie it all together!
DMT™ Attunement with Focus Technology!
Take Your Intention into the NEW Human Experience!

DMT™ Attunement

https://becomingbioquantum.com/DMT™Attunement

For more DMT™ Activations go to our YouTube Channel Becoming

BioQuantum: https://becomingbioquantum.com/YouTube

Notes

Notes

Glossary

ATP: Adenosine 5'-Triphosphate is the principal molecule for storing and transferring energy in cells. It is often referred to as the energy currency of the cell.

Advanced Human: 100% Human Potential. Body and Consciousness assimilate into Oneness. Body becomes DMT™ Intelligence. The 5th Light Body!

Bio-coded: Coding held in the body that holds Divine Intelligence.

Bio-Light: A state of being wherein the body holds expression, and the mind is held in Telethought or Source Intelligence. The Light spectrum brings color into the Darkness (black) through different focal points of the body without leaving Source Expression. You exist beyond Light yet use Light on a biological level to continue to shift 100% Consciousness into the body. You have the ability to sense different vibrations or Frequencies without ever leaving Pure Source Energy. This allows you to shift your environment or body as you continue to consciously meet 100% Intelligence…. until Consciousness is no longer needed.

Conscious Accelerator/Equilli: Ionic grid system that holds Consciousness in Source Expression and trains Consciousness to move beyond observation.

DMT™: Divine Molecular Technology, a Frequency that supports the Technology to turn on and hold expression of Source Intelligence.

Epigenetics: Study of gene expression as a result of your environment and/or of your behaviors. Observation of the loop.

Evolution Technology: Telepathic Technology that shifts Consciousness on a cellular level using DMT™ Frequencies. Awakens Intelligence within that decodes molecular technology or dormant DNA Codes. Foundation of the evolved human.

Gamify Reality: Access Source Intelligence outside of programming to reorder reality. Transcend form.

God Sphere: Represents looping cycle/programmed reality, the Matrix.

Home Frequency: The basic resonance you were born with. The Frequency of your High Heart.

Inside Out: To take something in the 3rd dimension or programmed reality and bring it into Source/DMT™ Intelligence, allowing everything to exist beyond time and space.

Ionic Grid: Ascended Ions click together creating a grid system. It is like electrical wires made of Light or a network of Frequencies hooking together to create a system that Source Intelligence runs through.

Lightbody: The conscious transition from density to Frequency. It is connected to Consciousness. Depending on what phase of the Lightbody you are in, you experience the body in different density or release of density.

Light Consciousness: The ability to hold Consciousness in Light or color of Light without leaving the Darkness. Pure Essence in expression without reflection. This will be your experience of the Ascended Body as Consciousness becomes 100% Human Potential. Color does not exist at 100% Potential; Light is not needed and creates loops in reflection. It is the ability to use Light in expression to shift density to a high spin state without leaving expression.

Matrix: Super Hologram or programmed reality that creates looping cycles or repeated patterns.

Mitochondria: Power houses of the cells. As cells transfer DMT™ Codes, mitochondria build in strength.

Negative Expression: DNA pulls in energy from the environment, first from the reality it "sees," then from the environment of the body/belly of the cell. It brings this expression or information into the DNA to create the body's reality or state of being.

Plasma Light: Ascended DNA expression held in the lifeline. Plasma Light is an organic system in a wave or electric state.

Positive Expression: DNA moves into the cell, body, and reality in expression of Source Frequency.

Pure Essence: A state of being in the purity of Source Intelligence at its highest state. Consciousness no longer exists. You are Essence beyond reflection of it. Pure Essence is the ability to be Source Intelligence without reflection. You are the Intelligence. You are form held in a space/time spherical creation. The first line of the Light Vehicle is created.

Quantum Body: The 4th Light Body. An experience beyond the programmed body. Holds Pure Intelligence stored in DNA/Source Intelligence.

RNA: A nucleic acid present in all living cells. Acts as a messenger carrying instructions from DNA for controlling the synthesis of proteins; in some viruses RNA rather than DNA carries the genetic information.

Singularity Divine Operating System: Ability to hold Consciousness in expression in the magnetic wave and create or operate from this state. To reconnect to the magnetic field, when you realize Consciousness has shifted to reflection, and move back into expression. The System is the connection of all three: Consciousness, magnetic field and expression linking to the experience of what is being created.

Super Hologram: The Matrix or programmed reality that creates looping cycles or repeated patterns.

Telethought: Thought within Source Intelligence.

Void: Empty space or Abstract Frequency. A space that holds Intelligence without form. Consciousness is held in emptiness until it attunes to the Intelligence held there.

Join the Movement

Website: https://jewelsarnes.com/
YouTube: https://www.youtube.com/@jewelsarnes
Instagram: https://www.instagram.com/jewels_arnes/

Coming Soon from Crossroads Publishing, LLC:
Book 2 of Becoming BioQuantum™

Get ready to journey beyond awareness and into cellular transformation with the next evolution in consciousness—**DECU: DNA Expression Cellular Upgrade**. This groundbreaking method empowers you to reprogram your cells, release outdated patterns, and fully experience the power of BioAscension™.

Through frequency, intention, and direct access to cellular processing, you'll activate your innate ability to ascend the limiting beliefs and programs held within your cells—awakening your body's infinite intelligence and remembering your true expression.

Learn more at Becoming BioQuantum™:
BecomingBioQuantum.com

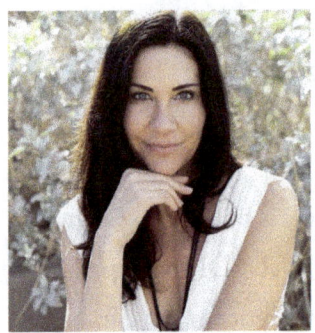

Jewels Arnes

Founder of Becoming BioQuantum™, Jewels is a visionary dedicated to advancing humanity through spiritual teachings and transformative products. With over 30 years of experience in Quantum Healing, she has crafted high-vibrational services and pioneered BioQuantum systems, shifting from molecular to Frequency-based healing. Jewels' unique ability to trace energy patterns helps uncover subconscious beliefs behind suffering, aging, and illness. Beyond her work, she enjoys hiking with her dog Roger and spending time with her daughters, while continually striving for physical and spiritual growth.

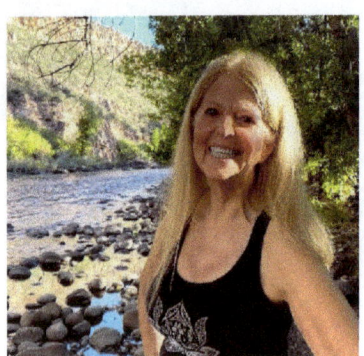

Cerena Lauren

Cerena has nurtured her connection with Spirit since childhood. She trained in healing modalities for over 40 years. Retired from a social services career and as a university professor, she holds an M.S.W. and a B.A. in Journalism. An accomplished writer and editor, she is a coach, peace minister, yoga instructor and a Bio-Quantum practitioner. Cerena is a dancer and enjoys photography and time with her son, Joshua. She has walked 5 Caminos of St. Francis in Italy.

www.ingramcontent.com/pod-product-compliance
Lightning Source LLC
Chambersburg PA
CBHW050854160426
43194CB00011B/2145